Core Training

For Greater Strength and Better Health

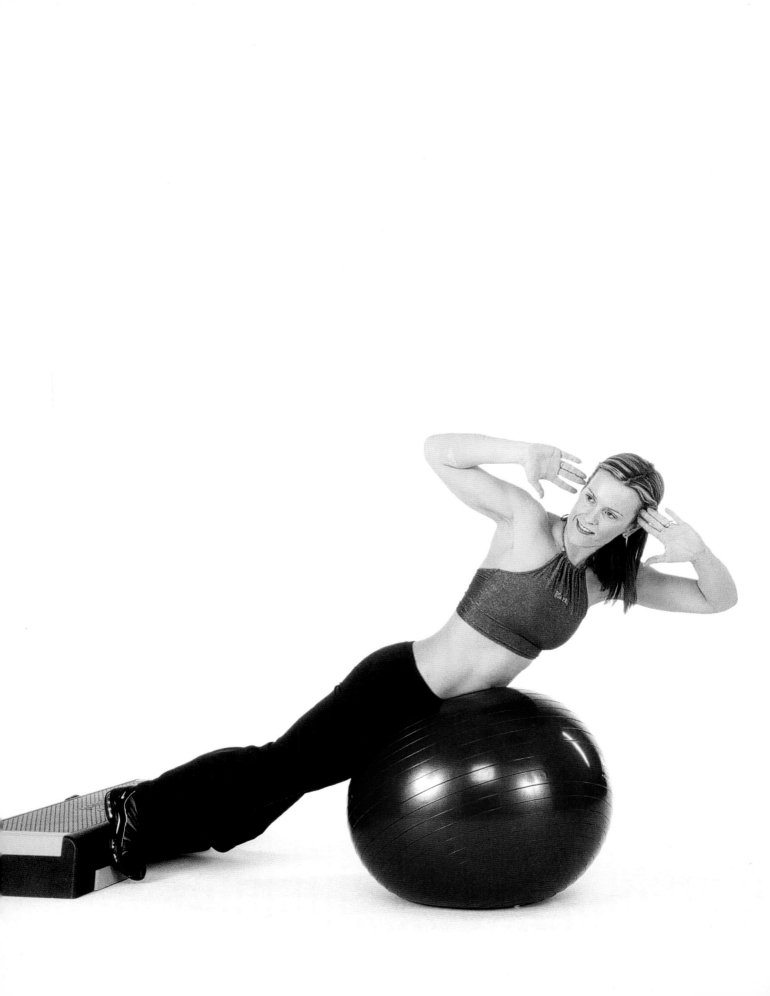

Core Training

For Greater Strength and Better Health

Thomas Boettcher

PRC

Produced in 2004 by
PRC Publishing
The Chrysalis Building
Bramley Road, London W10 6SP

An imprint of **Chrysalis** Books Group plc

This edition published in 2004
Distributed in the U.S. and Canada by:
Sterling Publishing Co., Inc.
387 Park Avenue South
New York, NY 10016

ISBN 1-85648-728-8

Printed and bound in Malaysia

AUTHOR'S ACKNOWLEDGMENTS

Core Training is the result of special insight and hard work. Thank you to: my brother Karl, for his core support;
my mother, a happy soul — good to the core; my father, whose core is consistency; T'ai Chi Master Raye Bemis,
whose thoughtful view of the core has truly earned her the title Master; James Milligan, the photography crew
and models, for bringing the book to life; HumanLabs and Infolocus associates, who correlate core data and wellness;
and all the trainers, physical education specialists, and medical professionals who have supported and endorsed
this work. You can explore health and wellness concepts further at humanlabs.com and infolocus.com.

The publisher wishes to thank Mike Prior for taking all the photography in this book,
including the photographs on the front and back covers. All photography is copyright © Chrysalis Images 2004

SAFETY NOTE
The exercises are for information only and are not intended to replace appropriate advice from a qualified practitioner.
Any persons suffering from conditions requiring medical attention should consult a qualified medical practitioner
before undertaking any exercises from this book.

Contents

Introduction

Most people have an appreciation for the role that general fitness plays in health and longevity, but find the solution to developing a totally fit and functional body somewhat elusive. Everyone knows that nutrition and activity is an important part of keeping fit and well, but how do you enable your body to function and perform at its optimum level?

The answer to achieving fitness and wellbeing is in developing the core part of your body, and this book will show you how to do that. What was once the hallmark of the elite athlete or prima ballerina is now the benchmark of fitness for every individual. Core strength and stability has meaning for all of us.

The core, in general, is defined as the central or basic part of a whole system—a foundation upon which you build. When speaking about your body, your core is the complex system of muscles, tendons and ligaments that comprise your body's foundation, roughly the area traditionally known as your trunk or torso.

What does this foundation do? It links the powerful movements of your upper and lower extremities, as well as maintaining internal organ function and acting as a life support system. Our core muscles stabilize us as we move or prepare to move our arms and legs. All movement originates at your core, hence it is your primary source of stability. Whether you're running, twisting, lifting weights, or picking up a suitcase, your core keeps your body stable and balanced.

What is core training?

Core training simply means exercising the muscles, tendons, and ligaments that connect your spine and pelvis area around the center of your body. It encompasses several aspects, most important of which are strengthening and stretching. Some muscles become weak from underuse and poor posture, while others become overworked and tight.

This imbalance in the body happens gradually as we succumb to everyday postural habits and challenges. It's not easy to maintain a healthy posture when computer screens and reading material cause us to bend our necks down, and sitting in one position for a long time leads to a slouching spine.

How do I benefit from core training?

You may imagine that the need for core training is most relevant for athletics, where precise coordination is needed for throwing, kicking, or running. But what about everyday life? The absence of core strength can lead to the common problem of backache, or injuries resulting from lifting simple items. This guide aims to help you gain the necessary core strength to avoid these injuries and aches and pains.

For all individuals, core training offers a higher level of general fitness. We will feel better and will notice that all of our daily activities seem easier. We won't tend to pull a muscle quite so quickly, perhaps a load won't seem so heavy, or we will generally function better throughout the week. An increase in muscle density will provide increased calorie burning capacity, which should also trim excess fat.

For athletes, core training gives more power to a swing or more distance in a throw, and they are not as prone to injury. Children will have healthier bodies, be able to move more dynamically, and will learn other athletic activities more quickly.

Those who are rehabilitating from a back injury will also benefit from core training, which will help to rebuild strength and protect against future re-occurrences. Pregnant women can tone their bodies not only for the physical ordeal of constantly lifting and moving extra weight during pregnancy, but also the challenge of giving birth and the many physical tasks they face afterward.

Seniors can build life and vitality into their best years. They can enhance stability and balance, which guards against potentially harmful falls. They can also guard against incontinence.

By following your own instincts and expending consistent effort, you will feel better, look better, function better, and protect yourself against everyday injuries, aches, and sprains.

Let's find our core

The area between your upper chest and the bottom of your torso defines your power center, the source of coordination and stability for your arm and leg movements. The most dynamic part of your core is the area from the bottom of your ribcage down to your lower pelvic region.

Your lumbar vertebrae provide the bone structure for this area, allowing for a highly flexible yet highly powerful transmission of power between your upper and lower body. The muscles, tendons, and ligaments of this core region provide stability and balance for your body in motion or at rest.

Let's take a tour of the muscle groups involved and get acquainted with what makes up the core. Your abdominals are composed of three muscle groups:

- **Rectus abdominus:** The set of long, vertical muscle tissue along the front of the abdomen that people associate with the "sixpack" or washboard stomach, which originates at the pubic bone.
- **Internal and external obliques:** Muscles that are located at the waist (side), and cross in the abdominal section to provide stability. Externals lie on the side and front of the abdomen, around your waist, while internals lie underneath, running in the opposite direction.

- **Transverse abdominals:** These run horizontally and are the deepest of the muscles for stability, wrapping around your trunk and spine for protection and stability.

Your abdominal muscles or abs work together for each exercise, but you can target each of the individual groups separately. Your very own "six pack" of rectus abdomins may even make an appearance once you reduce body fat, but that is just scratching the surface.

Your real foundation lies deep inside and includes the iliopsoas, intra-spinal, and pubococcygeal muscles that act as stabilizers and as a mechanism for transferring power:

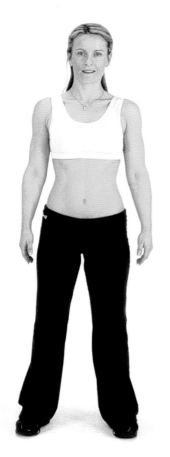

- **Iliopsoas:** The key to core power in a balanced and smoothly functioning body is the iliopsoas. This is a muscle group comprising the iliascus and psoas muscles.
- The **iliascus** muscle "fans" the pelvic anterior surface and connects with the psoas through a common tendon at the lesser trocanter. This means that it connects with your leg.
- The **psoas** muscle is a large hip flexor that plays a key role in creating the tensile strength that stabilizes the spine. There are two psoas muscles, one attaching on each side of the lumbar spine, starting at vertebrae T12 and directly linking the ribcage and trunk with the legs by running through the pelvis. The psoas helps transfer weight from the trunk to the legs and is counterbalanced by the obturators, a small group of muscles that attach within the pelvis. The psoas also enjoys a reciprocal relationship with the erector spinae and rector abdominis, working with your gluteal muscles for locomotion.

Your spine is superficially defined by your erector spinae, a set of three distinct muscles, and at a deeper level by the intra-vertebral muscles:

- **Erector spinae:** These provide longitudinal spine stability.

There are a group of superficial muscles of the **arms, shoulders** and **upper back** that surround the scapula (shoulder blades):

- **Levator scapulae:** Hold the scapula against the trunk.

- **Serratus:** Holds the scapula against the thoracic wall (chest area/upper part of the body).
- **Trapezius:** Muscles that draw back the shoulders and pull the head backward or to one side.
- **Rhomboids:** Hold the scapula against the thoracic wall.
- **Latissimus dorsi:** A broad, flat muscle on each side of the mid back area that allows shoulder adduction and extension.

The most often overlooked yet crucial link in the chain of core support is your perineum. This sheet of muscular fibers, known as the pelvic floor, is made of both interconnected voluntary and involuntary muscles. The most important muscular group within the perineum is Levator Ani, because it essentially sustains your various organs (the bladder, the vagina, the intestines, the uterus).

Alignment and posture

The most important principle of a core training regimen is the alignment of all the parts of your body. Alignment is the key word at a time when many of us perform sedentary tasks that allow us to slump or slouch while reaching our heads closer for information on computer screens and the pages of books. Core development requires that you strive to adhere to a strong functional alignment that counters the slouching habits of your normal daily life.

Part of the benefit of this guide is the repeated postural cues given as part of the exercises. Use that repetition to reinforce the movements, for functional alignment is a conscious act. Many refer to good posture as a "neutral" position; but just remember that alignment is an ongoing behavior that requires attention and deliberation.

Here are some guidelines for achieving alignment:

- Roll your hips under (this elongates the lower spine and allows the psoas to relax), as if you have a weight hanging from your tailbone pulling you down.
- Stretch up from the top of your head (this elongates the upper spine). Your chin is slightly tucked back.
- Press down in your underarms to further stretch the ribcage and spine. You will notice

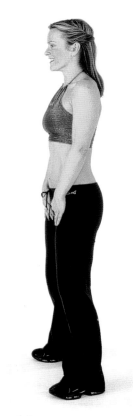

Aligned: Tucking under and elongating the spine gives functional alignment.

that this helps to "seat" the shoulders rather than allow them to be contracted upward by your levator scapulae and trapezius muscles.

- Gently pull your navel back away from your pants or shirt and toward your spine.

Breathing

In general, breathe out when you contract muscles and breathe in as you release, then relax and return to your original position. You actively work your abdominal muscles on your inhalation and exhalation, along with

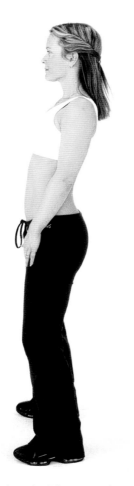

Unaligned: Note slight lower back hyperextension.

expanding and contracting your ribcage. Your ribcage is lifted through the effort of your underarm press, and you keep it centered over your pelvis by rolling your pelvis under and pressing back in your lower spine.

What to wear

When exercising your core area, you might benefit from wearing relatively tight-fitting clothing. This offers several advantages, both in function and form. For men and women, some degree of functional support and retention are necessary, especially for exercises involving the Swiss Ball. Functionally, you don't want loose or sliding clothing to disrupt or get in the way of your exercise.

We already know that alignment is a key aspect to the proper performance of each exercise. Therefore, each of us should try to check our body position and posture in a mirror during the exercise. If you don't have a mirror, maybe you can arrange to have a personal trainer or friend keep an eye on you.

Consult your physician

Consult your physician first to be sure you are medically prepared to try these exercises. Please check all the guidance you receive here against your own good common sense and prepare yourself with a medical checkup before initiating a program.

The content of this book is provided for informational purposes only, and is not intended to be a substitute for professional medical advice, diagnosis or treatment. Never disregard medical advice or delay in seeking it because of something you have read in this book.

Seek professional advice

Everyone's body is slightly different, and it helps to have a professional's opinion about the exact way in which you train your body and perform the exercises. Ask the opinion of someone you trust who understands physical training.

Keep a personal workout journal

Always record your workouts. Put a date and time on them. Record what you observe to know which workouts left you feeling great, and which ones left you feeling terrible.

As you embark upon your training regimen, create a workout journal or log that helps you track performance. This log can be as simple as a pencil and notebook diary or as comprehensive as a computer-based program that allows you to record sets, repetitions, aches and pains, and frequency of workouts. These can certainly come in handy when you wish to see which exercises have been effective for you and which have possibly caused discomfort, and the benefit is that you may track trends over time.

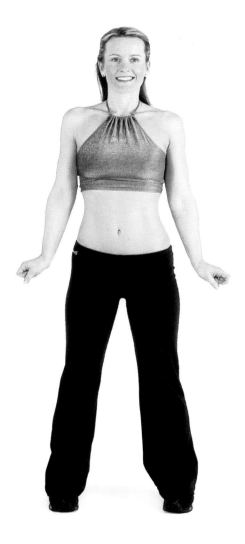

Equipment

- **Handweights/small dumbbells:** These should be easy to grip.
- **Ankle weights:** You can wear these weights around your ankles by using the Velcro closure.
- **Incline bench:** Check the stability of the base and the padding on the anchor.
- **Weight machine:** This should include the standard stacked weights and a cable system—specifically the apparatus necessary for lat pulldowns, rows, etc.
- **Roman chair:** For anchoring lower body and suspending the upper—you may substitute a padded table and partner to provide anchor.
- **Suspensory rack:** A freestanding rack with forearm pads for leg lifts—you may substitute parallel bars of any device that suspends the upper body and leaves the legs hanging free.
- **Medicine balls:** Normally supplied in a range of weights from 1–10lbs.
- **Staff:** A stretching pole—this should be as long as your arm-span.

- **Swiss ball:** The correct size allows you to sit with knees bent at a 90 degree angle.
- **BOSU** (1/2 swiss ball): A half ball mounted on plastic bottom or Reebok Core Board.
- **Step platform:** Needs to have an adjustable height, ensure that it will not slide out from underneath you.
- **Handled resistance band:** Typically color-coded degrees of resistance.
- **Nautilus:** Use this or any specialty machine or home device for crunches, flys, etc.
- **Exercise mat:** Keep it clean—you'll be spending some time on it.

Core training programs

Time management

Continue your cardiovascular routine, while you are exploring a new core training program. If you do not already have some method of increasing your heart rate at variable pace over time, find one. Core training should not detract from other vital fitness activities. Time is usually a constraint, so perhaps you could take a break from normal gym activities in order to exercise your core.

Designing a training program

The best training program for you is one you design for yourself with guidance. You must answer the basic questions of which exercises to perform and how frequently they should be performed.

Your program will emphasize stretching and range of motion initially; a "Core of Core" approach. Get the basics down and don't shock your body until it has a foundation of flexibility established. Then you can move on to a more comprehensive approach that entails trying all the exercises in the guide step by step. See the "Core of Core" suggestions in the table on page 15.

Daily practice

It is good to test yourself a little bit each day. However, the greatest threat to fitness and flexibility is injury. It is better to make gradual progress over a longer time period; everyone needs to exercise and move their body daily in some way.

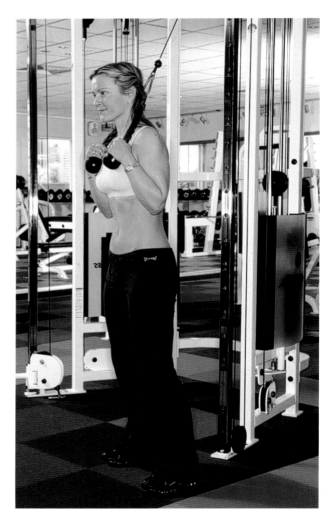

Sets and repetitions

Many people wonder how many repetitions or sets they should do. You should repeat the exercises with relative comfort in mind. Do not overstretch yourself. Aim for three sets of 8–12 repetitions. Start with only one if that is all you feel confident about doing. Do one repetition of a new exercise and get the feel of it. Then try two and aim to eventually try three. Coach yourself with just the right amount of patience and you will progress without suffering any injury.

Specialist groups

The following is a list of specialty groups that warrant special consideration in this guide:

- Pregnant women
- Seniors
- Those with back injuries and pain
- Younger athletes
- Elite athletes
- Healthy individuals

Remember that every individual is different; some progress rapidly and some progress slowly. Some injure themselves easier; some are more resilient. Common sense is your best guide for which exercises you undertake.

For seniors and pregnant women, the BOSU ball or balance board may not represent an acceptable risk, so these two may choose to develop balance skills while sitting on the Swiss Ball. Young and elite athletes start with good balance skills which may be readily enhanced by the BOSU or balance board. It is a matter of adapting functional need to acceptable risk levels.

Some will be able to handle any and all of the exercises regardless of condition, others will not. Try challenging ones gently and slowly at first. All back injuries are different, all pregnancies are different. You can test yourself and ask a personal trainer to join you as you make your own personal program.

Core influences

Training your core muscles will help correct postural imbalances, prevent injuries and develop efficient, functional movement patterns. Additionally, it will also activate your sensory awareness. This mind/body aspect of core training becomes clearer when looking at how martial arts have influenced it.

In general, the martial arts call upon the individual to harness the strength of the entire body. Noted for its graceful beauty and subtle power, T'ai Chi Chuan is a martial art with Daoist influences, stressing postural alignment. Its practice requires attention that is both inwardly focused and rooted in the environment.

Likewise, core influences can be found in the study of movement disciplines such as Pilates and yoga. Some types of yoga emphasize a long spine and are adequate for everyone. Pilates also increases core strength, endurance and lung capacity. These movement and alignment disciplines emphasize the functional necessity of core strength.

All athletic endeavors require core awareness. For instance, swimming calls for fundamental emphasis on core strength. Swimmers traditionally have strong, flexible core muscles because they must generate power from both arms and legs without the restriction of the ground. Stamina and power for long distance endeavors, such as extreme butterfly swimming in harsh open water, comes directly from the core.

How to use this book by group

Let's take a look at what a time-efficient functional program would look
like for an adult female or male, with standard fitness goals:

Beginners program

Elite, young, and healthy individuals can start with:

All Warm ups	Standing: Standard Step and Lunge
Supine: Abdominal Crunch	Standing: Free Weight Lunge
Supine: Oblique Crunch	Standing: Balanced Leg Extension
Supine: Elevated Leg Rotation	Swiss Ball: Swiss Kegels
Supine: Cross-legged Oblique Crunch	Swiss Ball: Rotations
Supine: Bridge	Swiss Ball: Contralateral Arm/Leg Extension
Supine: Bridge with Extension	Swiss Ball: Full Range Crunch
Floor Exercises: Bent Knee Side Crunch	Swiss Ball: Butterfly or Back Crunch
Floor Exercises: Bent Leg Side Crunch	Swiss Ball: Leg Raises
Floor Exercises: Jackknife	Gym Equipment: Crunch
Prone: Hip Extension	Medicine Ball: Trunk Rotation
Prone: Gluteal Crunch	Medicine Ball: Russian Twist
Standing: Pole	Warm Down Twists
Standing: Leg Adduction/Abduction	
Standing: Lunge	
Standing: Oblique Crunch	
Standing: Trunk Rotation	
Standing: Shallow Dead Lift	

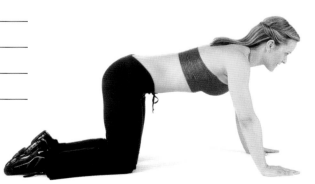

Intermediate/advanced program

Elite athletes and healthy individuals may progress to the full complement of exercises illustrated in this guide by following those exercises marked intermediate and advanced. Elite athletes will tend to work toward advanced exercises more rapidly and may seek greater weight and resistance levels in their exercises.

Seniors program

More than any other group, seniors may experience the most dramatic results from a core strength training program. Age tends to challenge muscle density, so seniors must pay specific attention to core muscles to maintain good posture and functionality.

Core of Core

Initially your program will emphasize stretching and range of motion. These are the basics:

All Warm ups

Kegels

Supine: Abdominal Crunch

Supine: Leg Lift with Compression

Supine: Leg Lift with Expansion

Supine: Oblique Crunch

Supine: Elevated Leg Rotation

Floor Exercises: Bent Knee Side Crunch

Floor Exercises: Bent Leg Side Crunch

Standing: Pole

Standing: Leg Adduction/Abduction

Standing: Oblique Crunch

Standing: Trunk Rotation

Standing: Standard Step and Lunge

Swiss Ball: Swiss Kegels

Swiss Ball: Rotations

Swiss Ball: Contralateral Arm/Leg Extension

Swiss Ball: Full Range Crunch

Swiss Ball: Butterfly or Back Crunch

Swiss Ball: Leg Raises

Gym Equipment: Crunch

Medicine Ball: Trunk Rotation

Warm Down Twists

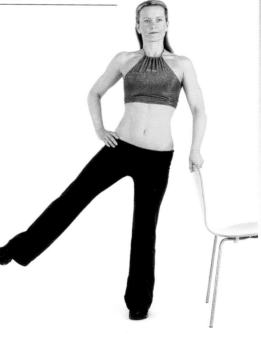

Warm Up

Always warm up first. Your body's connective tissue feels more elastic when your core temperature is elevated slightly. One of the best ways to get the blood flowing and elevate temperature is to walk. Swing your arms. Move your body simply. Flex your knees. Be careful not to begin static stretching exercises without first simply moving your body.

Warm Up Twists

Level: All

Suitable for: Healthy individuals

Unsuitable for: Back injuries

Area of concentration: Erector spinalis, abdominals

Start position: Stand with your feet slightly wider than shoulder width apart, eyes focused forward, arms relaxed at your side. Begin by imagining your spine as a straight cylindrical column.

Tuck your chin under and lift your head toward the ceiling from its crown (the very top of the head). Imagine you are being stretched upward by a rope attached to the crown of your skull. Allow your knees to flex and roll your hips under as you imagine the southern tip of your spine being pulled down by an attached weight. Open your hips so that your knees are vertically in line with your feet. Press forward at the fold of the hip joint, which is located at the front of the pelvis where your leg meets your trunk.

Pressing down in the armpits also seats the shoulders in a natural position so that levator muscles are not tugging them upward toward your head and tightening vertebrae along the way.

Exercise: Begin the twists by slowly rotating your waist around your spine, which should feel like a straight column, back and forth. Imagine your whole body rotating around a central vertical axis. Your arms should dangle loosely by your sides. Concentrate on the feeling of balance in your feet. Allow your arms to follow your waist as it twists slightly faster, however, never lead the movement with your arms. The arms should follow the core. Repeat for a slow count of 30, approximately 1 minute or until you feel loose.

End position: Slow your rotation and return to a standing posture. Your feet should be slightly wider than shoulder width apart, hips tucked under, knees flexed, and chin pressing back. Your spine should be long, your head up, and your tailbone down. Your arms should be relaxed at your side. Breathe through your nose in a relaxed manner.

Be aware: The twisting movement comes from turning the waist back and forth around the axis of the spine. Do not force the twist with surface muscles. Feel it originate from your core area.

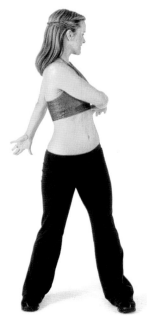

Warm Up Double Arm Stretch

Level: All

Suitable for: All

Area of concentration: Erector spinae

After you have twisted and moved your way to a loose and warm core body temperature, you can start to activate the muscles, ligaments, and tendons that you will be toning and strengthening. Begin with a double arm stretch up, which opens the chest and upper spinal area as well as the arms and allows your spine to elongate.

Start position: Start with your feet together, eyes focused forward, hands clasped in front of your face, and imagine your spine as a straight cylindrical column. You could vary this by unclasping your hands.

Exercise: Reach for the ceiling, remembering to keep your shoulders "seated" by pressing down in the armpits. Reach and release 8–12 times, breathing out on the way up and in as you bring your arms down.

End position: Return your arms to your side, hips tucked under, knees flexed, and chin pressing back. Your spine should be long, your head up, and your tailbone down. Your arms should be relaxed at your side. Breathe in a relaxed manner through your nose, feeling a distinct contraction and release of your abdomen muscles coupled with the expansion and contraction of your rib cage.

Be aware: Remember to press down at the heels and feel your weight on the ground while you simultaneously reach upward. This provides a good stretch for the spine.

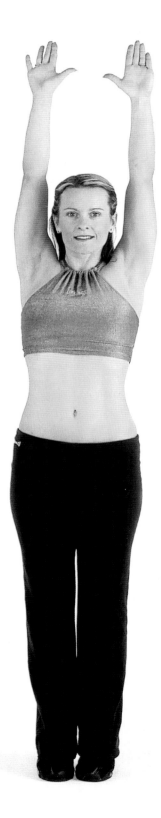

Warm Up Straight Leg Stretch Down

Level: All

Unsuitable for: Pregnancy, back injury

Area of Concentration: Glutes, psoas, erector spinae

In this exercise, while stretching your back, you will also have the opportunity to identify your hip joint and stretch the leg tendons and muscles that support you. The straight leg stretch mimics a seated position stretch of the same nature, yet it offers the added benefit of being a weight bearing position. This warmup includes the suggestion that you lock your knees in order to create straight legs. This helps to better stretch the hamstrings and related tissues. If you find locking your knees uncomfortable, try to make your legs as straight as possible and work slowly into the position as you gain flexibility.

Start position: Your feet are slightly wider than shoulder width, eyes focused forward, arms at the side.

Exercise: Bending at your hip fold, where your legs join your core, keep your spine straight, and bend as far toward a 90-degree angle as is comfortable. Reach straight down with your fingers touching back to back in repeated reach and releases. You could also bend down with your fingers outstretched, as shown here. Try 8–12 repetitions.

End position: Your feet should be slightly wider than shoulder width, eyes focused forward, arms at the side.

Be aware: You must keep stretching your spine straight and do not allow your neck to sag as you reach and stretch your arms and back. Bending comes from the hip joint only, just as if you were seated flat on the ground.

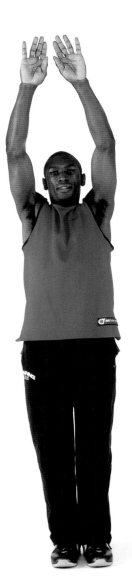

Warm Up Side Reach Oblique Stretch

Level: All

Suitable for: All

Area of concentration: Obliques, psoas, lower spine, glutes

Now you are ready to start more dynamic leg movements in association with core stretching. This weight shifting from leg to leg serves to enhance your balance and further elevates your body temperature.

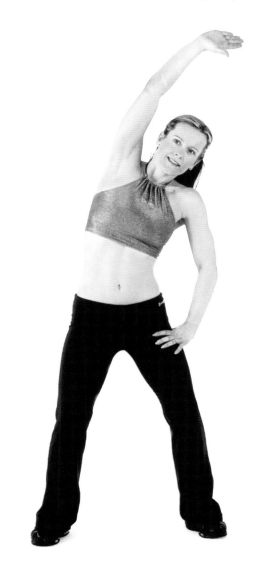

You will learn to feel grounded and adjust your posture and alignment in order to maintain balance. You will also learn to stretch dynamically rather than statically, a more realistic test for your body and mind.

Start position: Stand with your feet slightly wider than shoulder width apart and your eyes focused forward. Keep your knees bent, hips rolled under to elongate the spine as you flex at the hip fold, bend the right knee and place weight over the right leg.

Exercise: Pressing the right heel into the ground extend your left arm over your head. The left leg extends straight while the right leg bends. Feel the stretch along the left side of your body.

Retract the right arm and stand straight. Stretch the left arm up and stretch the other side of your body. Do 8–12 repetitions on each side.

End position: Your feet are slightly wider than shoulder width, eyes focused forward, arms at the side.

Be aware: Breathe out with every contraction, moving from the initial position to the stretch extension. Then relax the abdomen and inhale with every return to the initial position.

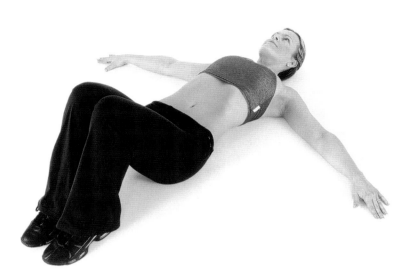

Double Lumbar Roll

▌ Level: All
▌ Suitable for: All
▌ Area of concentration: Abdomen, obliques, lower
lumbar spine

This is a fun stretching exercise that can work as a warmup or as an exercise. The use of a mat makes it a bit more comfortable. Those with back pain may want to try a single leg version first.

Start position: Lie on the exercise mat, keeping your spine long. Retract both legs to a 90-degree knee bend (or right angle, like a corner). Keep your feet flat, and your hands extended to your side for stabilization.

Exercise: Roll both knees over to the right very slowly, allowing the rest of your back to lift off the mat only to accommodate the pull of the legs. You should feel a stretch in your lower spine as the erector spinae release and elongate. As you keep your shoulder blades on the mat, roll both legs to the left side slowly and feel the stretch. Try this 8–12 times.

End position: Both legs rest on the mat.

Be aware: This movement is less effective if you swing your legs rather than move them slowly. Make sure you feel only a stretch and no sharp pain. Breathe easily and without holding through the repetitions.

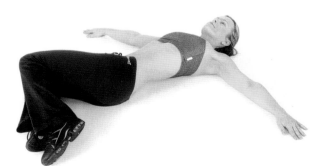

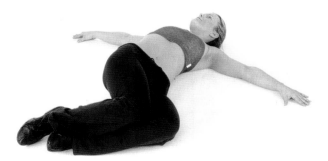

Cross Body Oblique/Glutes Stretch

Level: Beginner

Unsuitable for: Back injury, pregnancy

Area of Concentration: Psoas, glutes, lower spine

Seated stretching exercises allow you the opportunity to effectively isolate the hamstring/gluteal and erector spinae muscles without weighted pressure. Many basic hamstring stretches can be performed in a seated or standing position.

There are many variations of the basic seated "hurdler" stretch which may be substituted according to personal preference and background. This particular cross body stretch provides ancillary iliopsoas muscle benefits as well.

Start position: Sit on the exercise mat. Keep your spine long, and retract your right leg to a 90-degree knee bend. Keep your left leg out straight with your toes pointed up.

Exercise: Place your right foot flat on the mat to the left side of your left knee. Place your left arm to the right side of your right knee. Gently twist toward the right, pressing gently against your leg with your arm. Breathe out as you twist and hold.

Swap over your legs and repeat for the other side.

End position: Seated, both legs flat on mat.

Be aware: The stretch must be gradual and relaxed; do not force this stretch by levering your arm against your leg.

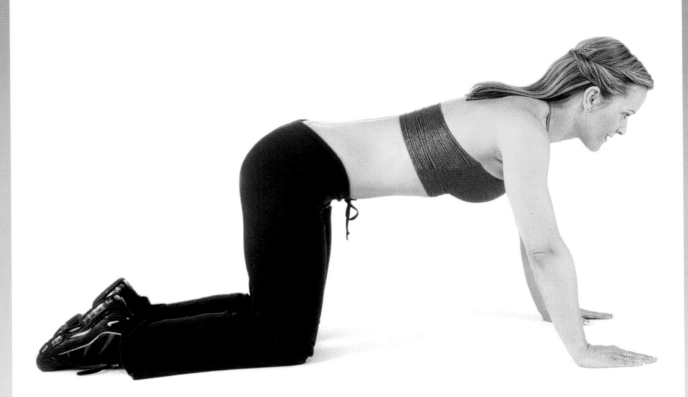

Frontal Lean and Retraction

Level: Beginner

Suitable for: All

Area of concentration: Abdominals, erector spinae

The frontal lean and retraction exercise allows you to dynamically explore your range of motion and slowly stretch yourself. You will see variations of this movement in dance classes, yoga studios, and pilates regimens. As long as you are careful with your knees, this should not present a problem for most individuals. Pregnant women may wish to be careful when stretching back and sitting on your legs. Go only as far as is comfortable.

Start position: From the prone position, face down on the floor or mat keeping your spine long and extended. Press yourself up on to your hands and knees to form a "tabletop" position, still facing downward. Your arms and legs resemble the four legs of a table, while your back forms the tabletop.

Exercise: Slowly shift your weight forward over your arms. Allow your muscles to extend for this movement.

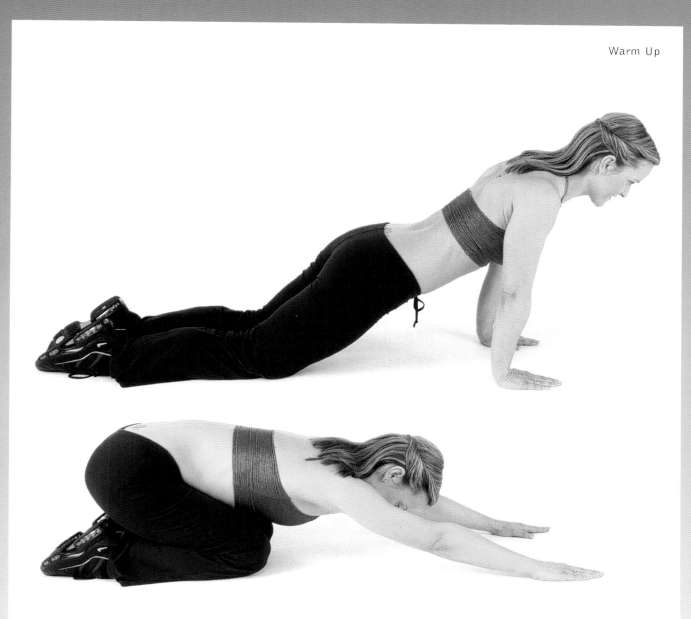

Next, slowly shift your weight all the way back to your legs, bending your knees to receive your body until you are as far back as comfortable. Your buttocks will move toward your heels as you stretch back.

Those with tender knees may want to be careful in choosing their range of motion for this movement. Go only as far as comfortable, feel the stretch, then return to center. Repeat 8–12 times.

End position: Resume the "tabletop" kneeling position. Your weight should be equally distributed

between your hands and knees. Breathe comfortably in this position and do not hold your breath.

Be aware: Remember to keep your spine long. Those of us with tender knees may wish to skip the mat version of this exercise and perhaps substitute a Swiss Ball stretch. The aim for a person in this situation is to avoid placing a "sheer load" on the knee joint, which stresses the anterior cruciate ligament. Continue breathing in a relaxed fashion throughout the exercise, assuring that you do not hold your breath.

Kegels Exercise

Kegels

Level: Beginner

Suitable for: All

Area of concentration: Pubococcygeal

Everyone wants to know the simplest starting point to core training. The easy answer is some sort of abdominal exercise. For those who really want to develop the core part of their body, they need to start at the very foundation. This is a terrific starting exercise for everyone — young, old, athletes, seniors, those with achy lower backs, and those with babies on the way.

We start with the pubococcygeal muscle. The pubococcygeal muscle, also popularly referred to as the PC muscle or the Kegel muscle, sustains the pelvic floor. The PC muscles stretch from the pubic bone in the front to the coccyx (tail) bone in the back.

The PC muscles lie beneath the surface of the very bottom area of our "trunks," supporting the pelvic organs like a hammock. Their identification and training are essential to good health and development of core strength. The maintenance of these muscles is vital to sustaining overall sexual health as well as control of excretory functions. In fact, this is the muscle that contracts in the moment of male ejaculation or female orgasm.

Because of the internal location of these muscles, men and women are perhaps unaware of the pubococcygeal's presence and importance to core strength. For women, the muscles provide support for internal organs such as the urinary tract, birth canal, urethra, uterus, and rectum. The muscles are essential for proper health during pregnancy and are utilized during childbirth and bladder control.

By why are they called Kegels? In 1948, gynecologist Dr. Arnold Kegel identified the pelvic floor. He realized that the simple exercise of contracting and relaxing the PC muscle resulted in muscle toning and increased volume, essentially becoming stronger and tighter. This strengthening and tightening exercise later was named after him. Done properly, Kegel exercises strengthen weak PC muscles and strengthen the foundation in our quest for a stronger core.

Start position: The first step in performing a kegel is to first identify what it is you are actually working on. You can't contract the right muscles if you don't know where they are. The simplest and most direct way is to do a simple test: interrupt the flow of urine. The muscles used to do this in women or men are the PC muscles. Be careful not to tense the stomach, buttocks, or thigh muscles as they can take over from the PCs.

To do the exercise, lay down on your back in a comfortable position with your entire spine elongated and as much of it touching the ground as possible. Make sure all your muscles feel relaxed and you are looking straight up at the ceiling. Place your feet shoulder width apart and bend your knees to a 90-degree angle (or right angle, like a corner), with your hands down by your side.

Exercise: Contract your PC muscle and hold that contraction for three seconds. Remember to continue to breathe normally and maintain relaxation in all the surrounding muscles. This may not be so easy in the beginning. Relax the PC muscle.

End position: At the end of the repetition of contraction and relaxation, stay calm and relaxed on your back, noticing that you haven't used your buttocks muscles or your abdomen muscles. Try another repetition, up to eight, remembering to be specific with the PC muscle group only.

Be aware: For most people it takes more that two weeks to notice results, but be sure to maintain the integrity of the exercise by not over-forcing and causing the larger surrounding muscle groups to interfere. You want to work the PC only with this exercise. We'll get to the other ones next.

Intermediate: As you become more comfortable with the exercise, you may increase your set number to three and your duration of contraction hold.

Advanced: Vary your hold time, with short tension/release times then long, as you contract on a Swiss Ball.

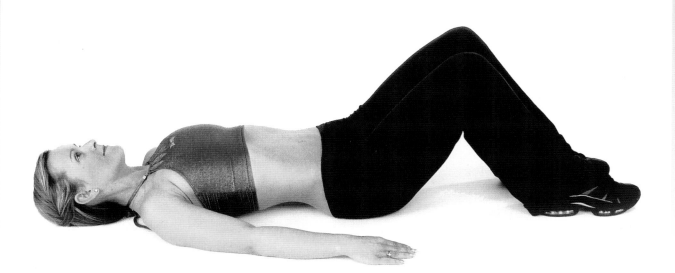

Supine

Double Legged Roll Back

Level: Beginner

Unsuitable for: Pregnancy, back injury

Area of concentration: Lower spine

The Roll Back is a fun exercise that can work as a warmup or exercise. Use of a mat makes contact on the spine easier. Be sure that you don't use momentum to complete this exercise.

Start position: Lie on the exercise mat, keeping your spine long. Retract your legs to a 90-degree knee bend (or right angle, like a corner). Keep your feet flat and your hands relaxed over the upper chest or shoulder joints.

Exercise: Keeping your shoulder blades on the mat, tuck your knees toward your chest, and roll your hips up and toward the ceiling. You will feel yourself roll back. Hold the upright position of your legs for a second, then slowly lower them back to the mat.

End position: Both legs rest on the mat.

Be aware: This movement is less effective if you swing your legs rather than move them slowly. You may also tuck tightly during your roll.

Abdominal Crunch

Level: Beginner
Suitable for: Healthy individuals
Unsuitable for: Prenatal
Area of concentration: Abdominals

Doing a crunch correctly requires a measure of patience. Experience suggests that it is extremely challenging to isolate the abdomen muscles if you are tempted to grab the head and strain your body to lift. For this reason, crossing your arms across your chest removes the temptation for the crunch to turn into a neck-pulling exercise.

Start position: Lie on the floor or a mat, facing the ceiling, with your spine comfortably relaxed and touching the surface along its entire length. With your feet flat on the ground and shoulder width apart, flex your knees to a right-angle position. Roll your hips under to elongate your lower spine. Relax your arms and hands on your chest, with palms facing downward. Breathe comfortably.

Exercise: Contract your abdomen muscles until you lift your shoulder blades off the ground. Keep your lower back flat and do not lift it off the mat. Concentrate to thrust your chest toward the ceiling while your chin stays tucked in. Hold at the top of the movement for two seconds and squeeze your muscles. Lower yourself slowly back to the mat. Repeat this eight times.

End position: Lie flat keeping your spine long and abdominal muscles relaxed.

Be aware: In the enthusiasm and strain of the exercise, it is often tempting to lift the chin toward the ceiling as part of the overall exertion. Resist this urge and only lift your shoulder blades as high as you can by using your abdominal muscles. Breathe as regularly as possible throughout the exercise. Each contraction of the abdomen muscles should correspond with an exhalation, while each relaxation should correspond with an inhalation.

Intermediate: Use an incline bench.

Advanced: Use a free weight resting on your upper chest, or stand using an overhanging stretch cord or cable machine weights.

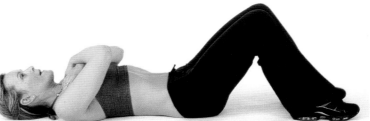

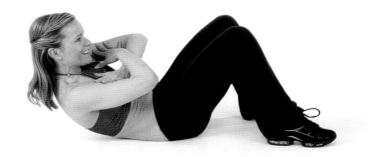

Oblique Crunch or Side Crunch

Level: Beginner

Suitable for: Seniors and prenatal

Area of concentration: Obliques

The side crunch is a very stable way to work your obliques, while protecting your spinal position. As always, care is necessary to assure that you don't pull up with your neck, as curiosity induces you to sneak a peek at your feet. Looking isn't necessary. Feeling the obliques do some toning work is necessary.

Start position: Lie on the floor or a mat, facing the ceiling. Your spine should be comfortably relaxed and touching the surface of the floor along its entire length. With your feet flat on the ground and shoulder width apart, flex your knees to a 90-degree angle position (or right angle, like a corner). Roll your hips under, creating a tucking feeling as you elongate your lower spine. Keep your arms and hands comfortably relaxed, palms down beside you. Breathe in and out comfortably and don't hold your breath.

Exercise: Contract your right side muscles to draw your upper body down toward your feet as you remain lying on your back. Feel the sensation of reaching with your right hand toward your right foot in the muscles at the side of your body. Allow the exercise to be driven not by your arm muscles, but from your side. Maintain a long spine throughout the motion. Now release and return to the start position, then repeat the process to your left side. Hold at the end of each crunch for a second, squeeze your oblique muscles, then actively release that squeeze and allow them to freely elongate as you crunch over to the other side.

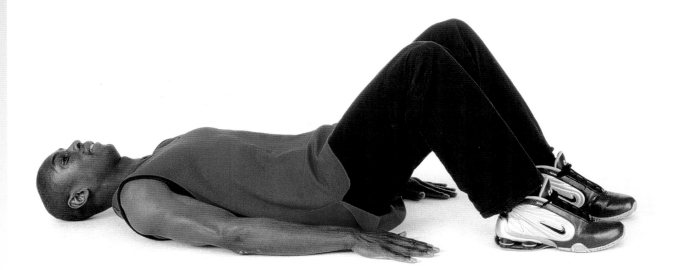

End position: Lie flat with an elongated spine with your abdominal muscles relaxed.

Be aware: In the enthusiasm and strain of the exercise, it is often tempting to lift the chin toward the ceiling as part of the overall exertion. Resist this urge and keep your chin tucked in. Breathe as regularly as possible throughout the exercise.

Intermediate: The best intermediate version of this exercise is done with stretch cords and is described in the standing stretch cord exercise.

Advanced: Elite athletes may wish to try a standing version of this exercise with free weights, as described in the free weight section.

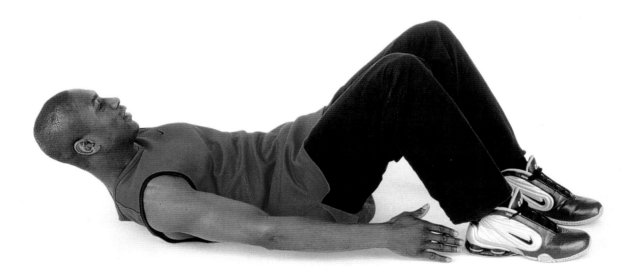

Bridge

Level: Beginner

Suitable for: Healthy individuals

Unsuitable for: Back injuries

Area of concentration: Transverse abdominis, lower spine

This exercise strengthens the supporting muscles and tendons of the pelvic region.

Start position: Lie on the floor or a mat, facing the ceiling, with your spine comfortably relaxed and touching the surface along its entire length. With your feet flat on the ground and shoulder width apart, flex your knees to a right-angle position. Roll your hips under to elongate your lower spine. Relax your arms and hands at your side, releasing any tension in your abdominals, and breathe comfortably.

Exercise: Keep your gaze fixed on the ceiling, gently contract your gluteals, and feel your heels press into the ground as your hip joint moves toward the ceiling.

Imagine your pelvic crease—the two lines where your abdomen joins your legs—reaching for the ceiling, as you allow your hip joints to relax and open. Once you have reached a comfortable end to your range of motion, begin to slowly lower yourself back to the floor, gradually releasing your muscles.

End position: Lie flat on the ground or mat, eyes to ceiling and arms at your side.

Be aware: Keep your scapulae (essentially your shoulders) and spine flat during the exercise. Resist the urge to look at your feet during the movement. Continue to breathe naturally, without holding your breath during any portion of the exercise.

Intermediate: Extend one leg as you form the bridge.

Advanced: Secure a free weight plate on your chest with a strap (so that it doesn't slide down your chest in the bridge position and hit you in the chin). Alternatively, use a Swiss Ball as a foundation.

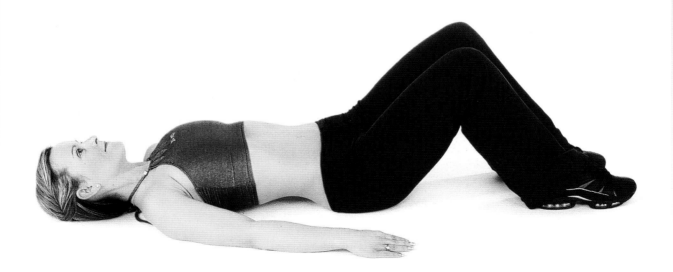

Bridge with Extension

Level: Beginner

Suitable for: Healthy individuals

Unsuitable for: Back injuries

Area of Concentration: TA, psoas

Building upon the base provided by the bridge, you can add more stability and balance skills to your exercise.

Start position: Lie on the floor or a mat, facing the ceiling, with your spine comfortably relaxed and touching the floor along its entire length. With your feet flat on the ground and shoulder width apart, flex your knees to a right angle position. Roll your hips under to elongate your lower spine. Relax your arms and hands at your side as you release any tension in your abdominals and breathe comfortably.

Exercise: Keeping your gaze fixed on the ceiling, gently contract your gluteals, feeling your heels press into the ground as your hip joint moves towards the ceiling. Allow your hip joints to relax and open.

Once you have reached a comfortable end to your range of motion, begin to slowly transfer weight to your left foot on the ground, and extend your right leg straight. Lower the right leg to the ground, then shift your weight to the right foot and extend the left. Upon completing the desired repetitions of this exercise, lower yourself back to the surface, feeling your muscles relax. Try eight repetitions.

End position: Resume the flat on the ground or mat position, eyes to ceiling and arms at side, ready for another repetition if desired.

Be aware: Keep your scapulae (essentially your shoulders) and spine flat during the exercise. Resist the urge to look at your feet during the movement. Do the exercise deliberately and slowly, developing stability and control.

Intermediate: Try securing a free weight plate on to your chest as in the Bridge exercise.

Advanced: Try a Swiss Ball as a foundation.

Elevated Leg Rotation

Level: Beginner
Suitable for: Seniors and prenatal
Area of concentration: RA, psoas

Many exercises that strengthen core stability also heighten your awareness of the deeper muscles that govern your spinal alignment and posture. This is one of those exercises that is shared by pilates enthusiasts and calls upon you to use both the rectus abdominus surface muscles and the deep psoas muscles. The iliopsoas musculature largely governs our stability, from simple walking around to high stress weight and direction change in elite athletics, or extra weight

bearing during pregnancy. In this case we are learning to release and relax the psoas.

Start Position: Lie on the floor or a mat, facing the ceiling, with your spine comfortably relaxed and touching the surface along its entire length. With your legs flat on the ground and toes up, roll your hips under to elongate your lower spine. Relax your arms and hands with your palms down beside you. Breathe in and out comfortably.

Exercise: Pulling in your front abdominal muscles (rectus abdominus), while your back stays flat, lift your left leg toward the ceiling and attempt to keep it as

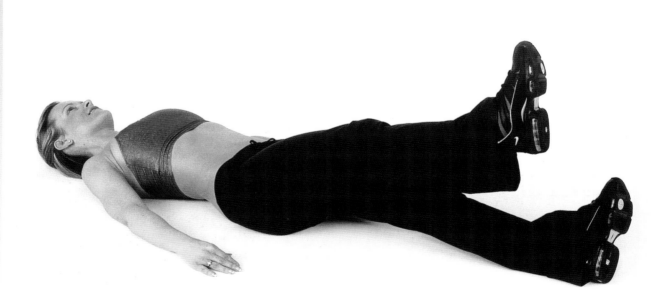

straight as possible while pointing your toe toward the ceiling. Rotate your left leg once in a clockwise direction, making a circle as big as your foot. Rotate once in the opposite direction.

Slowly lower your left leg to the ground, returning to your ready position. Repeat this process with the right leg, working up to eight repetitions for each leg.

End position: Lie flat and elongate your spine. Relax your abdominal muscles.

Be aware: It is better to only lift your leg as far as you can go without bending it, just gradually pointing the toe higher and higher as you gain awareness of your psoas muscle and learn to release it. Breathe as regularly as possible throughout the exercise.

Intermediate/advanced: This exercise may be made more challenging with the addition of a soft ankle weight affixed around each leg.

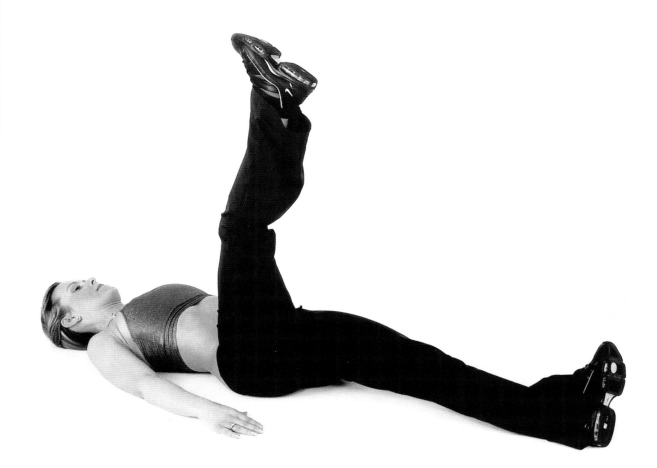

Cross-legged Oblique Crunch

Level: Beginner

Suitable for: Healthy individuals

Unsuitable for: Prenatal, back injury

Area of Concentration: Obliques

The Cross-legged Oblique Crunch offers you the opportunity to add some subtle refinement to your core. By crossing your legs, you lengthen the pelvic region.

You will see many different hand positions associated with the Crunch, which are all fine and can add or subtract from the degree of difficulty. However, experience suggests that it is extremely challenging to isolate the obliques if you are tempted to grab the head and strain your body to lift. For this reason, you should cross your arms over your chest to remove the temptation to turn the Oblique Crunch into a neck-pulling exercise.

Start position: Lie on the floor or a mat, facing the ceiling, with your spine comfortably relaxed and touching the floor along its entire length. With your feet flat on the ground and shoulder width apart, flex your knees to a right angle position (90 degrees, like a corner). Roll your hips under to elongate your lower spine. Cross your left leg over your right one. Relax your arms and hands over your chest, with your palms facing downward right below your neck. Breathe in and out comfortably.

Exercise: Contract your abdomen muscles until you lift your shoulder blades off the ground. Your lower back should stay flat and not lift off the mat. Twist, using your oblique muscle until your right shoulder is aimed toward your left kneecap. There is no need to actually try to touch the kneecap.

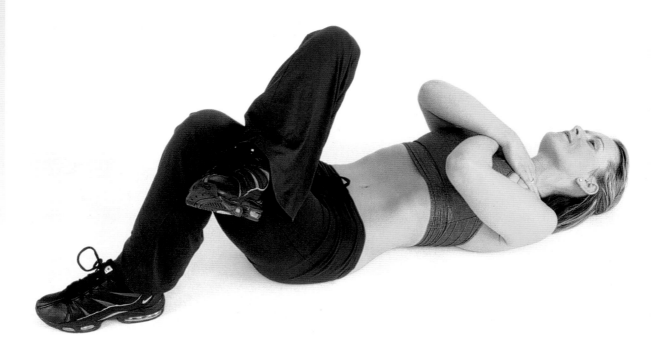

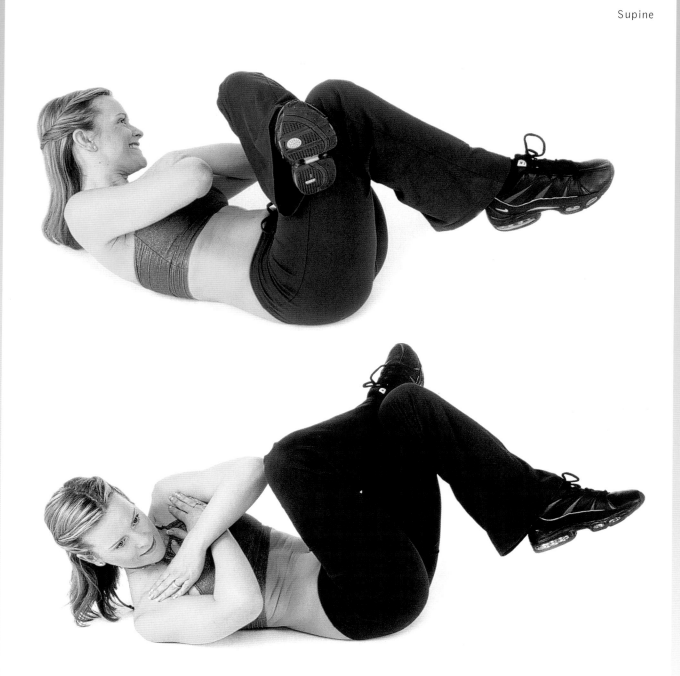

Hold at the top of the movement for a second and squeeze your muscles. Lower yourself slowly back to the mat. Repeat this motion eight times, then reverse your leg cross and do the exercise for the left side.

End position: Lie flat with an elongated spine and with your abdominal muscles relaxed.

Leg Lift with Compression

Level: Beginner

Suitable for: Healthy individuals

Unsuitable for: Prenatal

Area of Concentration: Adductor, iliopsoas, and pubococcygeal

This is a special exercise that requires a little extra concentration. This flexion exercise concentrates on the adductor and pubococcygeal area, while addressing the psoas. The special nature of this exercise lies not so much in what is being done externally, but instead focuses on what you are doing internally.

In essence, the Leg Lift with Compression is a ground-based interpretation of the suspensory rack exercise done with a squeezable ball or pilates ring between the knees and ankles.

The key to the effectiveness of this exercise is its Kegel-based focus. While you are squeezing the ball and lifting your knees toward your chest, keep your focus on the contraction of your pubococcygeal muscle group (Kegel muscles).

Start position: Lie on the floor or a mat, facing the ceiling, with your spine comfortably relaxed and touching the surface along its entire length. With your feet flat on the ground and shoulder width apart, flex your knees to a right-angle position (90 degrees, like a corner). Roll your hips under to elongate your lower spine. Relax your arms and hands on your chest, with your palms facing downward below your neck. Breathe comfortably.

Place a small-sized Swiss or other squeezable ball between your knees and apply pressure.

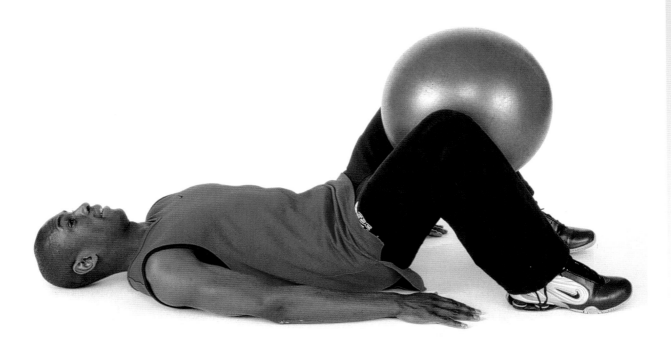

Exercise: Bend from your hip joints as you lift your knees towards your chest. You should experience a flexing sensation at the point where your leg joins your core body. Be sure to keep your hips rolled under and do not allow your lower spine to arch. Hold that position, then slowly release the legs back to the straight-down position.

While completing the repetition, remember also to contract your Kegel muscles, the pubococcygeal group, while squeezing together with your knees. Do eight repetitions, then repeat the exercise with the squeezable ball between your ankles.

End position: Lie flat with an elongated spine and relax your abdominal muscles.

Be aware: Remember that your spine, especially your lower spine, should stay as flat as possible against the mat. Do only as many as you can while maintaining this proper form, and discontinue if you feel strain on your lower back. Breathe as regularly as possible throughout the exercise. Each contraction of the abdomen muscles should correspond with a leg lift, while each relaxation should correspond with a return to extended leg.

Intermediate: Add ankle weights to your legs.

Advanced: Perform the exercise with a medicine ball.

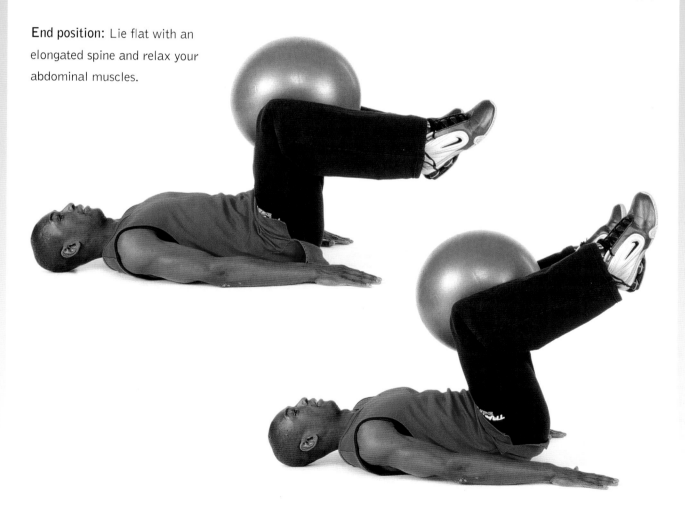

Leg Lift with Expansion Against Cord

| Level: Beginner
| Suitable for: Healthy individuals
| Unsuitable for: Prenatal
| Area of Concentration: Abductor, iliopsoas,
| and pubococcygeal

This flexion exercise concentrates on the abductor and pubococcygeal areas, while addressing the psoas. It provides balance and harmony to a comprehensive group of muscles such as the iliopsoas, the glutes, and those around the abdomen region.

The Leg Lift with Expansion Against Cord is a ground-based interpretation of the suspensory rack exercise done with stretch cord around the knees and ankles. You will be doing the same maneuver here, except that you will be on your back. The key to the effectiveness of this exercise is its Kegel-based focus. While you are expanding the cord and lifting your knees toward your chest, concentrate on contracting the pubococcygeal muscles. The result is a very dynamic core strengthening exercise.

Start position: Lie on the floor or a mat, facing the ceiling, with your spine comfortably relaxed and touching the floor along its entire length. With your feet flat on the ground and shoulder width apart, flex your knees to a right-angle position (90 degrees, like a corner). Roll your hips under to elongate your lower spine. Relax your arms and hands on your chest, with palms facing downward below your neck. Breathe in and out comfortably. Place an expandable cord around your knees and apply pressure.

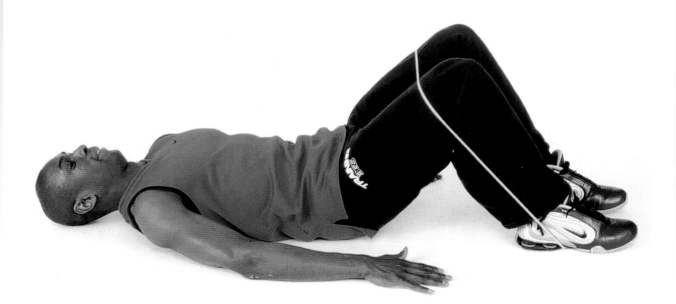

Exercise: Bend from your hip joints as you lift your knees towards your chest. You should experience a flexing sensation at the point where your leg joins your core body. Be sure to keep your hips rolled under and do not allow your lower spine to arch. Hold that position, then slowly release your legs back to the straight-down position.

While completing the repetition, remember also to contract your Kegel area muscles (the pubococcygeal group), while expanding your knees against the restraint of the cord. Do eight repetitions.

End position: Lie flat keeping your spine elongated and your abdominal muscles relaxed.

Be aware: Remember that your spine, especially your lower spine, should stay as flat as possible against the mat. Do only as many as you can while maintaining this position, and discontinue if you feel strain on your lower back. Breathe as regularly as possible throughout the exercise. Each contraction of the abdomen muscles should correspond with a leg lift, while each relaxation should correspond with a return to an extended leg.

Intermediate: Add extra cords to your legs.

Advanced: Add ankle weights to your legs.

Floor Exercises

Jackknife

Level: Intermediate/advanced
Suitable for: Healthy individuals/elite athletes
Area of concentration: Upper abdominals

Much has been said of the stresses and strains various Jackknife positions place on the body, yet many swear by it. There are ways to make it more approachable.

The Jackknife series of exercises call upon the body to do strenuous work. The upper abdominals are targeted, but too much pull can hyperextend the lower spine because of a reaction in the iliopsoas muscles. For that reason, start with a one-legged version of the Jackknife and build from that platform.

Be sure that your shoulders remain in a "seated" position by pressing down in your armpits. Your upper back should be smooth, as your scapulae lie flat and in line with your spine.

Start position: You may begin with your upper body either on the mat or 45 degrees in the air; the same goes for both legs. If you start in the air, your body should look like a "V." If you start on the mat, you should look flat.

Exercise: A standard jackknife can be completed by "crunching up" to a closed position, bringing the upper body and the legs toward each other. Leave your hands crossed over your chest or extend them to reach toward your feet, still keeping your shoulders seated. Whether you perform your Jackknife motion from the V position or from the flat position, try not to bounce into your next repetition. Try eight repetitions.

An easier version of the exercise is to leave one leg bent at 90 degrees and on the mat, and leave the other leg straight. Try eight repetitions.

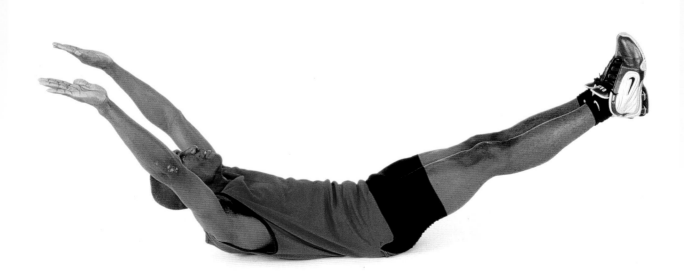

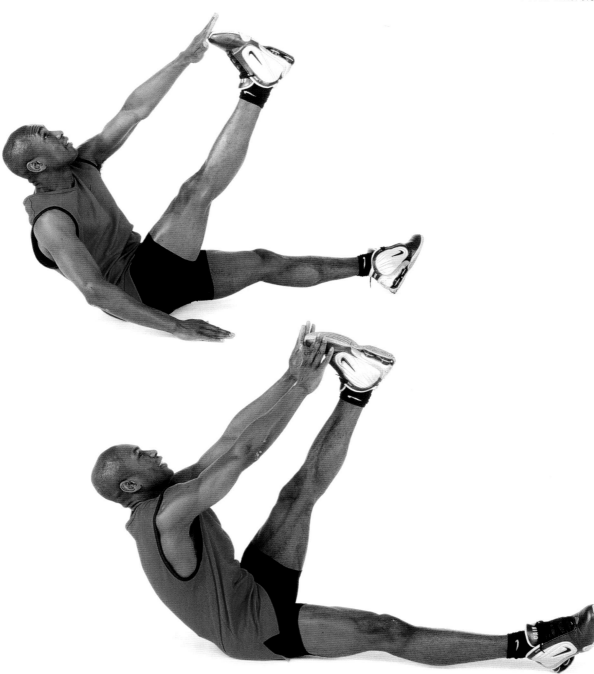

End position: Sit in a "V" position, or lie flat on the mat.

Be aware: Be careful that you keep your spine elongated and your shoulders seated. You want your exercise effort to come from your core, so keep your chin tucked in. Breathe out as you contract and inhale as you release throughout the exercise. Be certain that you feel no strain on the lower back.

Bent Knee Side Crunch

Level: Beginner

Suitable for: Seniors and prenatal

Area of concentration: Obliques

This exercise is simple and concise. It doesn't need much space or dramatic movement, but you do need to concentrate your effort.

Start position: Lie on one side of your body with your knees flexed to a 90-degree angle. Cross your hands and cover your shoulders as you straighten your spine. Keep your eyes forward.

Exercise: Contract your oblique (side muscles) to draw your upper body off the mat. Remember that you are releasing opposite side muscles to allow for your trunk to lift. Now return to start position, repeating

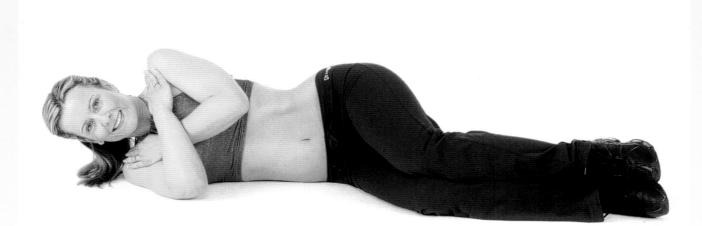

the exercise eight times. Hold at the end of each crunch for a second, squeeze your oblique muscles, then actively release that squeeze.

End position: Lie on your side with your abdominal muscles relaxed.

Be aware: Breathe as regularly as possible throughout the exercise. It is very tempting to use the back muscles in this exercise. Be careful to isolate the area you intend to exercise.

Intermediate: Use stretch cords as described in the Standing section of this book.

Advanced: Elite athletes may wish to try a standing version of this exercise with free weights, as described in the Free Weight section.

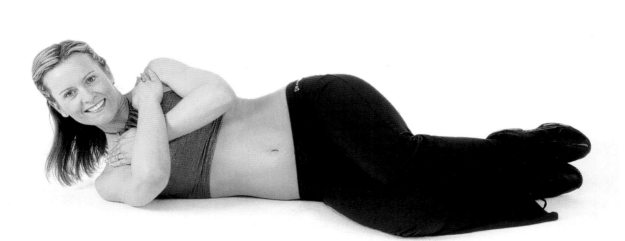

Bent Leg Side Crunch

Level: Beginner

Suitable for: Seniors and prenatal

Area of concentration: Obliques, adductors, abductors

Once you have decided to work your obliques from your side, you might as well get your legs moving too.

Start position: Lie on one side of your body with your legs stretched straight below you. Bend your lower leg to a 90-degree angle in order to stabilize your body from rolling over. Cross your hands and cover your shoulders as you straighten your spine. Keep your eyes looking forward.

Exercise: Contract your oblique (side muscles) to draw your upper body off the mat, releasing obliques on the opposite side to allow for the lift. Simultaneously, lift your same side leg off the mat and hold. If you wish to further test your balance, try the same movement with the underlying leg straight. You may even try lifting both legs at the same time or lift the underlying leg to the upper leg.

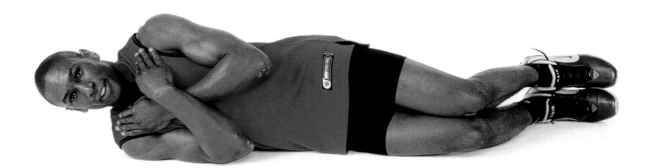

Now release and return to the start position, repeating eight times. Hold at the end of each crunch for a second, squeeze your oblique muscles, then actively release that squeeze. Roll over and try the other side.

End position: Lie on your side with your abdominal muscles relaxed.

Be aware: Breathe as regularly as possible throughout the exercise. It is very tempting to use the back muscles in this exercise. Be careful to isolate and use the muscles you want to exercise.

Intermediate: The best intermediate version of this exercise is done with stretch cords and is described in the Standing section of this book.

Advanced: Elite athletes may wish to try a standing version of this exercise with free weights, as described in the Weights section.

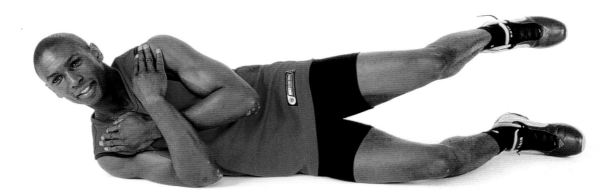

Prone

Hip Extension

Level: Beginner

Suitable for: Healthy individuals

Unsuitable for: Those with sore knees

Area of Concentration: Erector spinae, gluteals, psoas

The Hip Extension is a simple exercise for exploring the strength of muscles and tendons that stabilize your lower spine and help you to stand erect, walk vigorously, and sit with good posture. You will find variations of this movement in almost any discipline, from yoga to martial arts to basic warmup routines for track and field.

Start position: From the prone position, face down on the floor or mat with an elongated spine, press yourself up to a hands-and-knees "table" position still facing downward. Maintaining balance, shift the weight to your left leg and extend the right leg straight back until you have formed one long line from your head, down your spine to your heel. Your hips remain tucked under to help maintain this straight line.

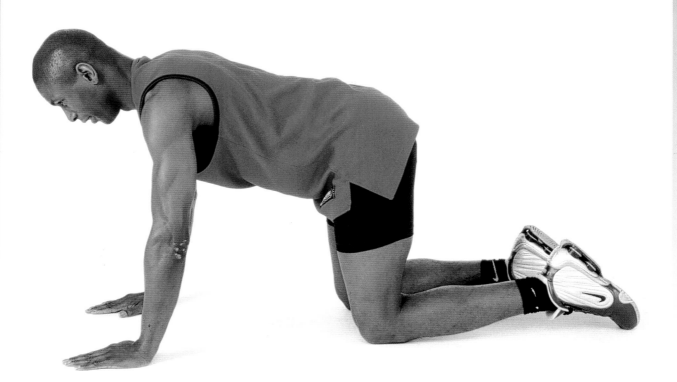

Exercise: Continue to fix your gaze at the ground, contract your gluteal and hamstring muscles, while keeping your lower back relaxed and straight. Raise the leg as high as is comfortable, then slowly lower it to 1 inch (2.5cm) above the ground. That is one repetition. Repeat the up and down motion for your desired number of repetitions, then change legs.

End position: Resume the "table" kneeling position with your weight equally distributed on all four hands and knees, breathing comfortably.

Be aware: Remember to keep your spine elongated. Those with tender knees may wish to skip the mat version of this exercise and perhaps use a Swiss Ball as a foundation and do a double leg lift. The aim is to avoid placing a "sheer load" on the knee joint, which stresses the anterior cruciate ligament. Breathe comfortably, and do not hold your breath.

Alternative/intermediate: Use a Swiss Ball as a foundation to do a double leg lift.

Advanced: Do a standing exercise with a stacked weight machine.

Gluteal Crunch

Level: Intermediate

Suitable for: Elite, youth, normal

Unsuitable for: Seniors, prenatal

Area of Concentration: Erector spinae, intra–vertebral muscles, gluteals

This type of exercise is sometimes known as the Superman. You may find that this exercise is more comfortable and effective, if you raise your body off the ground with one to three mats. This removes possible strain on your lower back and allows for a greater range of motion in the exercise.

Start position: Lie in a prone position with your face down on the floor or mat. Make sure your spine is elongated by tucking in your chin and rolling under your hips. Extend your arms in front of you. Your legs should lie straight back. If possible, arrange your mat so that your core is supported but your legs and arms hang off to the side.

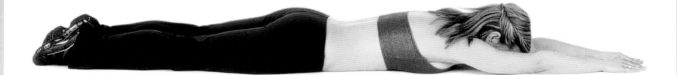

Exercise: With your head still facing down, lift your arms, upper body and legs off the mat. Hold that position for a count of three while your back and gluteal muscles remain contracted. Slowly release to lower your arms and legs back to the mat, then repeat eight times.

End position: Resume the relaxed prone position with an elongated spine.

Be aware: Remember to keep your spine elongated. Continue breathing in a relaxed fashion, assuring that you do not hold your breath as you balance your weight on your abdominal muscles.

Alternative: Try the Uni- and Contralateral Crunch exercises on page 50.

Advanced: Try the Superplank exercise on page 51.

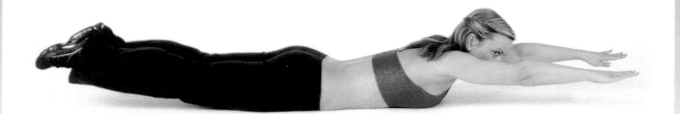

Uni- and Contralateral Gluteal Crunch

Level: Intermediate
Unsuitable for: Pregnancy and back injury
Area of concentration: Erector spinalis, gluteals

After you have mastered the Gluteal Crunch exercise, you will be ready to introduce variation to the core muscles that support your spine and hips. Rather than lift all arms and legs at once, you can practice coordination and balance.

Again, you may find that this exercise is more comfortable and effective if you raise your body off the ground with one to three mats. This allows for a greater range of motion in the exercise and possibly relieves some hyperextension in the lower lumbar region when lying in a flat prone position.

Start position: Lie in a prone position with your face down on the floor or mat. Make sure your spine is elongated by tucking in your chin and rolling under your hips. Extend your arms in front of you. Your legs should lie straight back. If possible, arrange your mat so that your core is supported but your legs and arms hang off to the side.

Exercise: To do the Unilateral Gluteal Crunch, lie with your head facing down and lift your left arm, upper body, and left leg off the mat. Hold that position for a count of three while your back and gluteal muscles remain contracted. Slowly release to lower your arm and leg back to the mat, then repeat with the right arm and right leg, eight times for each.

To do the Contralateral Gluteal Crunch, lift the left arm and upper body along with the right leg. Hold that position for a count of three. Release slowly and repeat for the right arm and left leg combination.

End position: Resume the relaxed prone position with an elongated spine.

Be aware: Remember to keep your spine elongated. Continue breathing in a relaxed fashion, assuring that you do not hold your breath as you balance your weight on your abdominal muscles.

Intermediate: You may add strap-on ankle and wrist weights to further challenge the body.

Advanced: Try the Superplank exercise opposite.

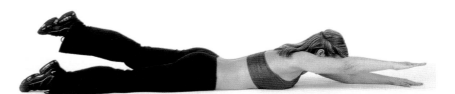

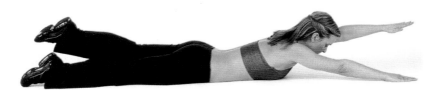

Superplank

Level: Advanced

Suitable for: Healthy individuals

Unsuitable for: Pregnancy

Areas of Concentration: Iliopsoas, abdominals (rectus and transverse), erector spinae, gluteals, pubococcygeals

Here's a combination exercise developed specifically to mimic the demands of what many consider the toughest physical activity known to humanity — swimming the butterfly. This exercise's combined range of motion works the front and back core muscles, encouraging balance and strength.

Start position: Face down on the floor or mat and elongate your spine by tucking your chin in and rolling your hips under. Extend your arms in front of you and your legs straight back.

Exercise: With your head still facing down, lift your arms, upper body, and legs off the mat. Hold that position for a count of three while your back and gluteal muscles remain contracted.

Now bring your arms in beside you, forearms resting on the mat with your hands next to your shoulder and elbows fully bent, toes pressing into the ground. With your hips tucked under, arch your entire spine as if someone had a rope attached around your waist and was lifting you from the ceiling. You are basically pressing your whole body up while resting your weight on your toes and forearms.

Slowly lower yourself back down to the ready position for the next crunch, with your arms and legs extended.

End position: Resume the relaxed prone position with an elongated spine.

Be aware: Remember to keep your spine elongated. Continue breathing in a relaxed fashion, assuring that you do not hold your breath as you balance your weight on your abdominal muscles. Breathe out during the crunch and the arch, and breathe in slowly as your release these positions.

Alternative/advanced: You may add strap-on ankle and wrist weights to further challenge the body.

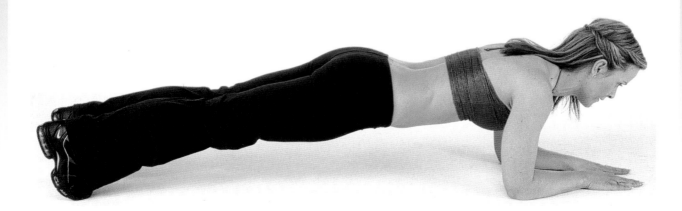

Standing

Standing Pole

Level: All
Suitable for: Everyone
Area of concentration: All core support

The Standing Pole exercise is so simple and so deliberate that anyone can do it, yet everyone can spend a lifetime trying to master it. Standing Pole is a discipline of Yi Quan influenced by T'ai Chi.

Standing Pole encourages a quiet mind which lends itself to the task of internal reflection and introspection. This is not some passive relaxation technique, however. Standing Pole is a rigorous and challenging physical discipline that requires active participation and constant reassessment of alignment, effort, and internal feedback. The trick is actually to continue the exercise while expending less and less exertion. One of the nicest features of Standing Pole is that it is appropriate for everyone—seniors, pregnant women, those with back injuries, as well as athletes.

Done in the proper fashion, this exercise creates a feeling of "groundedness" and solid core development. It may seem like a leg exercise, but don't let that fool you. Success in core strengthening comes primarily from the ability to identify and reach those deep muscles that provide stability and long term power. Standing Pole gives everyone the chance to reach a little deeper and tone muscle groups such as the iliopsoas that are so vital to true core stability.

Start position: Wear shoes with flat soles, socks or stand in bare feet. Stand with your feet slightly wider than shoulder width apart. Bend your knees slightly, flex comfortably at hip joint, with your abdomen relaxed. Tuck your hips in for support and to elongate your spine. You will feel your weight sink down onto your feet with pressure on your heels.

Press down in your armpits to extend your upper spine upward, feeling the crown or tip of your head reaching for the ceiling, while your chin stays tucked in.

Exercise: Imagine that you approach a pole and want to wrap your arms and legs around it while still standing. Your action is similar to that of someone hugging a large tree trunk. Try it. Keep your shoulders seated, meaning down, and reach around with your arms. Now relax as many muscles as possible and try breathing in and out from your abdomen and chest, expanding and contracting for inhalation and exhalation.

You have slight flexion at your hip joint, your knees are bouncy and flexible and your arms hug your imaginary pole at around chest height (sternum). You are reaching you head toward the ceiling and your spine is long and as straight as you can stretch it. Be sure to keep your hips rolled under and do not allow your lower spine to arch. Hold this position for as long as is comfortable, then relax.

End position: Standing comfortably with an elongated spine, gaze forward and relax your abdominal muscles while maintaining the posture described above. At the moment you weaken, relax away from the exercise and shake out your legs.

Be aware: Throughout the exercise, you must keep your hips rolled under and chin tucked in. Breathe as regularly as possible throughout the exercise, making note of the areas within your core that feel tight or relaxed. Take note of which movements allow you greater flexibility or expansion of your core. Experiment with balance. Feel your feet and look for your weight to sink lower as you identify deeper core muscles and surrender control of surface muscles.

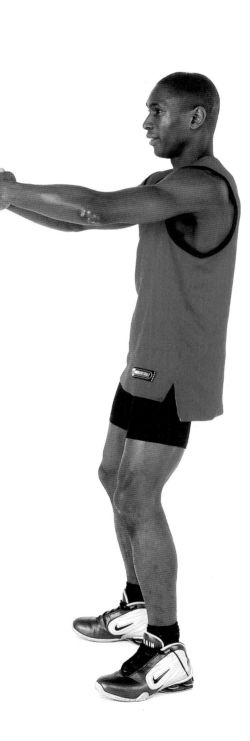

Leg Adduction/Abduction

| Level: Beginner
| Suitable for: All
| Area of concentration: Iliopsoas, gluteals, adductors, abductors

One of the simplest ways to loosen and extend the muscles of the core is to find your adduction and abduction range of motion. Adduction of the leg is simply medial movement towards the midline of the body, whereas abduction is medial movement away from the midline of the body. Why is it important to our core capabilities? Core muscles work in harmony to provide us with stability, flexibility, posture, and locomotion. We involve the muscles of our core when we call upon the abductors and adductors to do their job. Adduction is accomplished with adductors brevis, longus and magnes, whereas abduction is accomplished with gluteus medius and minimus. However, you also must release and lengthen your psoas in order for these muscles to work properly. If you really want to test your core balance, try these without the stabilization of a wall, chair, or bar.

Start position: Stand in front of a wall, bar, or chair with feet about shoulder width apart and one hand stabilizing you against the wall or chair. Your hips should be rolled under, your knees slightly bent, shoulders down, and your heels pressing into the ground.

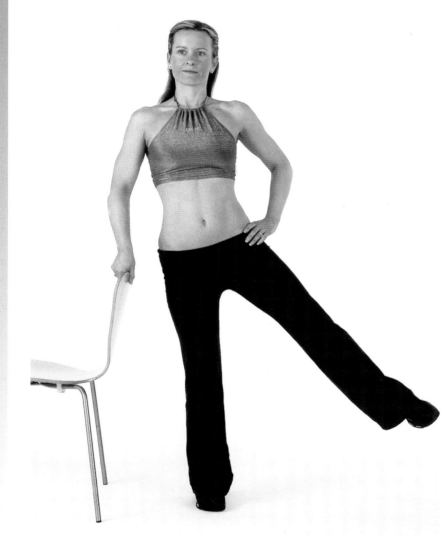

Exercise: With your right leg slightly bent, make a sweeping motion across the front of your body and back. Repeat eight times and then do the same for the left leg.

End position: Stand comfortably with your spine elongated, and your feet shoulder width apart. Look forward and relax your abdominal muscles.

Be aware: For stability, be sure that you feel your weight pressing into your heel on the standing leg. Keep your spine long and your torso relatively straight up and down during the sweep as you feel your abdominals stretch. Throughout the exercise, you must keep your hips rolled under and chin tucked in. Breathe as regularly as possible throughout the exercise.

Intermediate: You can make this more difficult with ankle weights.

Advanced: You may perform this with cable and stacked weights.

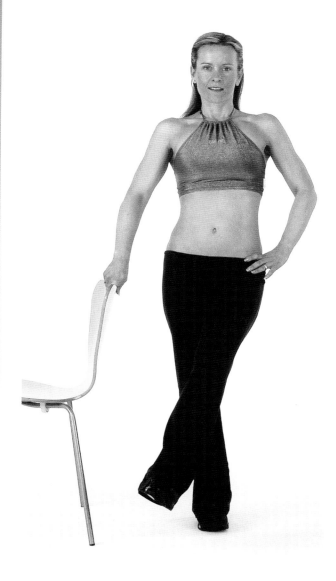

Standard Step and Lunge

■ Level: Intermediate/advanced
■ Suitable for: Healthy individuals, athletes
■ Unsuitable for: Seniors, back injury, prenatal

The step is a great piece of equipment for training your core. If you walk up a few flights of stairs in addition to fine aerobic conditioning, you also have a perfect opportunity to work your core muscles.

By keeping the discipline of tucking the hip joint and activating the iliopsoas and pubococcygeal muscles, you reinforce good posture and call upon the erector spinae and abdominals to do their work. Typically, the step platform is deployed in some sort of aerobic workout setting. Everyone can work standard step exercises in order to enhance their core. The

lunge adapts particularly well to the step, offering variety and an increased degree of difficulty.

Start position: Stand with your feet about shoulder width apart, step placed in front of you at slightly longer than normal stepping distance. Your hips should be rolled under, knees slightly bent, shoulders down, and heels pressing into the ground.

Exercise: With your right foot, make a step onto the step. As you gain confidence, you may place the step further away. Allow the right leg to lower you slowly

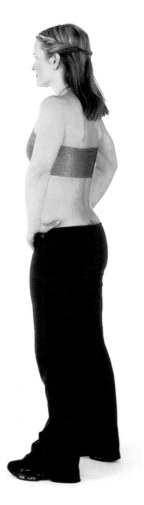
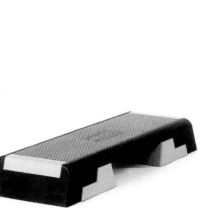

down until your upper thigh is parallel to the ground. Sink only as low as is comfortable. Your back foot, the left, should roll up on to your toes to allow this lunge step. Your left knee may tap the ground. Push back up with the right foot as you tuck the hip and feel the core muscles working for you. Raise yourself up and step back to your standing position, then repeat with the left leg leading into the lunge. Try eight on each leg.

End position: Stand comfortably with an elongated spine, feet shoulder width apart. Look forward and relax your abdominal muscles.

Be aware: For stability, be sure that you feel your weight pressing into your heel on the lunging foot. Keep your spine long and your torso relatively straight up and down during the lunge. Throughout the exercise, you must keep your hips rolled under and chin tucked in. Breathe as regularly as possible throughout the exercise.

Advanced: You may add free weight resistance.

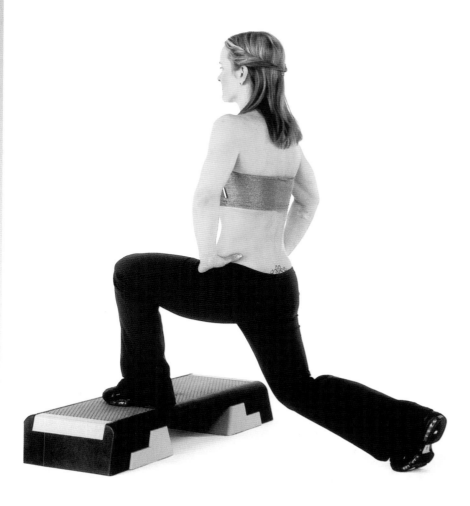

Free Weight Lunge

- Level: Intermediate/advanced
- Suitable for: Healthy individuals/athletes
- Unsuitable for: Seniors, back injury, prenatal

Once you have mastered the standard Step and Lunge, you may wish to increase the difficulty with the addition of free weights. The action of the exercise remains the same, and the emphasis on straight posture remains key to working your core muscles.

Start position: Stand with feet about shoulder width apart, weights on either side of your feet and the step in front of you at a distance a little further than normal stepping length. Your hips should be rolled under, knees slightly bent, shoulders down, and heels pressing into the ground. Pick up the weights without making your spine slump, keep your eyes forward and your chin tucked in.

Exercise: With your right foot, make a step that feels slightly longer than normal, yet is not uncomfortable. As you gain confidence, you may place the step further out. Allow your right leg to lower you slowly down until your upper thigh is parallel to the ground. Sink only as low as comfortable. Roll up onto your toes on your back foot, the left, to allow this lunge step. Your left knee may tap the ground.

Now push back up with the right foot as you tuck the hip and feel the core muscles working for you. Raise yourself up and step back to your standing position,

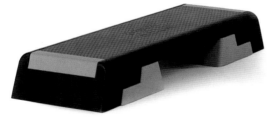

then repeat with the left leg leading into the lunge. Try eight on each leg.

End position: Standing comfortably with your spine elongated, and your feet shoulder width apart, gaze forward with your abdominal muscles relaxed.

Be aware: For stability, be sure that you feel your weight pressing into your heel on the lunging foot.

Keep your spine long and your torso relatively straight up and down during the lunge. Throughout the exercise, keep your hips rolled under and chin tucked in.

Breathe as regularly as possible throughout the exercise and don't hold your breath.

Advanced: You may add additional free weight resistance.

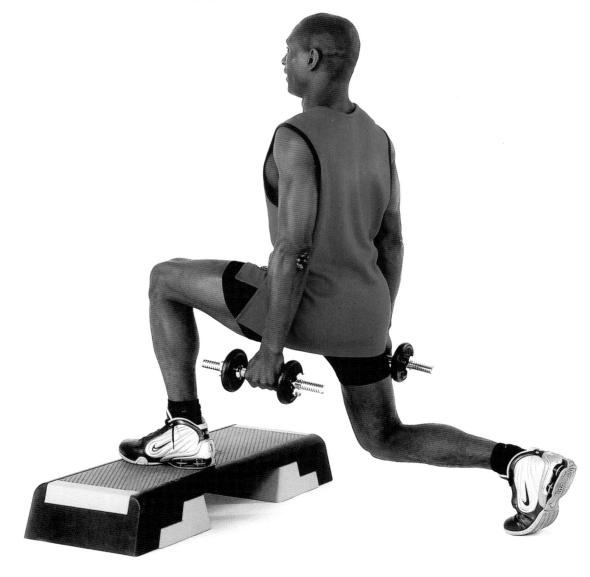

Oblique Crunch

Level: Intermediate/advanced
Suitable for: Healthy individuals, athletes
Area of concentration: Obliques

The Standing Oblique Crunch allows you to use gravity to enhance the subtle balance mechanisms at work in your pelvic area. As always, maintaining a correct posture is essential in order to benefit properly from this exercise.

Start position: Stand on top of the handled resistance cord, feet about shoulder width apart, with equal length of cord extending on each side. Your hips should be rolled under, knees slightly bent, shoulders down, and your heels pressing into the ground.

Pick up the handles without making your spine slump, keep your eyes forward, and your chin tucked in. Stand straight up with the resistance handles pulling on the band on both sides.

Exercise: Begin by contracting the oblique muscles on your right-hand side and allowing the obliques on your left-hand side to extend. Be sure that your hips are tucked under and your knees remain flexed. Hold that side crunch for three seconds, then return to standing straight up, and stop for one second. Repeat for the opposite side, and aim for eight repetitions of each side, feeling the work in the obliques and hip muscles.

End position: Stand comfortably with an elongated spine and look forward with your abdominal muscles relaxed.

Be aware: Throughout the exercise, you must keep your hips rolled under and your chin tucked in.

In the enthusiasm and strain of the exercise, it is often tempting to lift the chin toward the ceiling as part of the overall exertion. Resist this urge and keep your chin tucked in. Breathe as regularly as possible throughout the exercise.

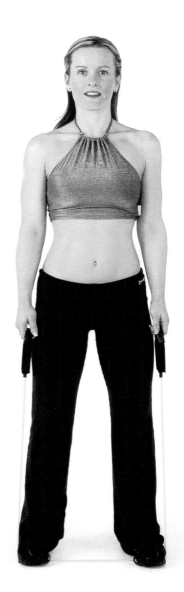

Intermediate: You may increase the difficulty of the exercise by shortening the cord or pulling higher with your hands, increasing the tautness.

Advanced: Athletes may wish to try a standing version of this exercise with free weights, as described in the Weights section.

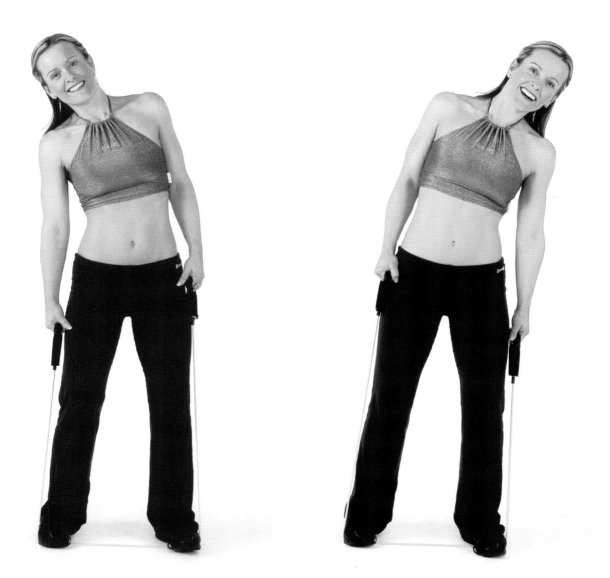

Pull Down Crunch with Cord

Level: Intermediate

Suitable for: Healthy individuals, athletes

Area of concentration: Abdomen, iliopsoas

This exercise requires a little care in setting up, but it is a useful variation on the crunch and adds the dynamic of corded resistance and activation of the iliopsoas because of the standing position. Be careful not to strain the lower spine, as for any other crunch exercises working the abdomen.

Start position: Stand underneath a suspended horizontal bar, feet about shoulder width apart, legs straight. Your hips should be rolled under, shoulders down, and heels pressing into the ground. The handled stretch cord should hang over the horizontal bars. Hold each handle over your underarm/shoulder area as you bend 90 degrees at your hip joint (pelvic fold) and prepare to use your abdomen muscles.

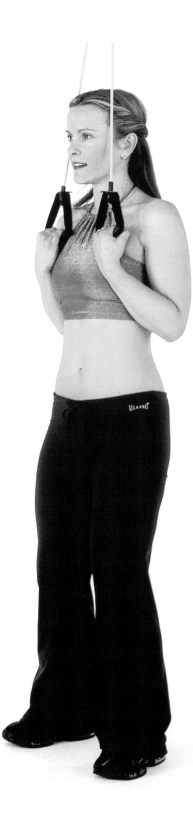

Exercise: Contract your abdomen muscles only in order to pull down the stretch cord. By keeping your legs straight, you will experience a stretching in your hamstrings. You may also bend your knees slightly, but keep the discipline of a straight back and be sure to use only your abdominals for your range of motion.

End position: Finish with your legs bent 90 degrees at your hip, your spine straight, and breathing comfortably.

Be aware: You are working only the upper abs in this exercise, so breathe out upon contraction and inhale upon release.

Intermediate/advanced: You may shorten the length of the cord or double up cords.

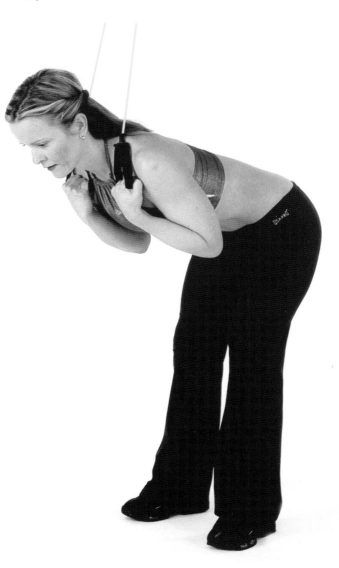

Trunk Rotation

Level: Intermediate

Suitable for: All

Area of concentration: Erector spinalis, obliques, transverse abdominals

When you are ready to really work the core of your body, and use the erector spinalis muscles as well as the obliques and transverse abdominis, then it is time to use a resistance band or cord. By performing the trunk rotation against the stretching resistance of the cord, you will extend and strengthen the internal muscles of the core.

Start position: Anchor your stretchable cord by looping it around a fixed exercise bar or other secure fixed device about waist high. Stand with your left side facing the anchor. Hold the two handles in your right hand and steady yourself by standing with your knees slightly flexed and feet shoulder width or a little further apart. Stand so that the resistance is engaged when you stretch the cord until your right hand is holding the handles on your right side.

You may hold your hand slightly away from your hip in a fixed position.

Your hips should be rolled under, shoulders pressing down, and heels pressing into the ground.

Exercise: Breathing out, turn your trunk to the right side, feeling pressure against your left leg. Slowly allow the stretching resistance to turn you all the way back,

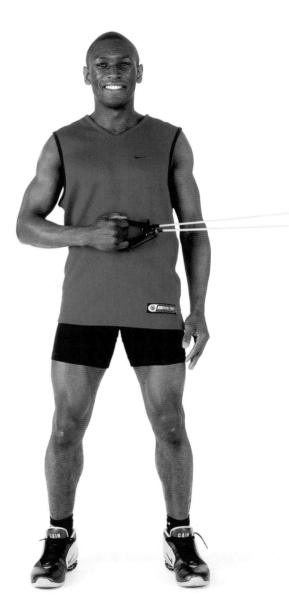

completing one rotation. Try this eight times then switch position to your other side.

End position: Standing comfortably with an elongated spine, feet shoulder width apart, look forward with your abdominal muscles relaxed.

Be aware: For stability, be sure that you feel your weight pressing into your heel on the pushing leg. Keep your spine long and your torso relatively straight up and down during the rotation as you feel your abdominals stretch.

Throughout the exercise, you must keep your hips rolled under and chin tucked in. Breathe out on contraction and in on return.

Advanced: You may perform this with a cabled stacked weight system.

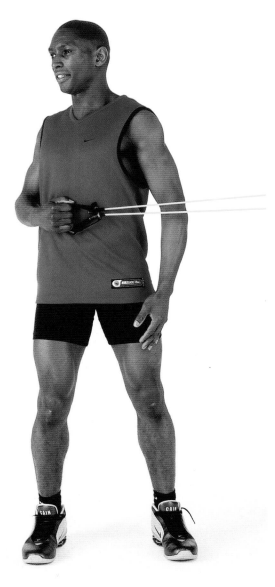

Shallow Dead Lift

Level: Intermediate

Suitable for: Young people, athletes

Area of concentration: Psoas, glutes, all core support muscles

The handled resistance cord is a great way to add difficulty to your core workout without progressing directly to free weights. Done in the proper fashion, this exercise creates a feeling of "groundedness" and solid core development. It may seem like a leg exercise, but don't let that fool you, you are still working your core muscles.

Again, care must be taken here not to stress the knee joint while working against the resistance of gravity and the stretchable cord. Keep your knees bent slightly and your spine straight.

Start position: Stand on top of the handled resistance cord, feet about shoulder width apart, with equal length of cord extending on each side. Your hips should be rolled under, knees slightly bent, shoulders down, and heels pressing into the ground.

Pick up the handles without slumping your back. Keep your eyes forward, and chin tucked in. Stand straight with the resistance handles pulling on the band on both sides.

You may vary this exercise by keeping your legs straight, but be very careful not to strain your lower spine and ligaments.

Exercise: Bend from your hip joints as the cord provides resistance. Be certain that your knees do not extend forward further than the vertical line rising straight up from your toes. You should experience a flexing sensation at the point where your leg joins your core body. Be sure to keep your hips rolled under and do not allow your lower spine to arch.

Next, slowly press your heels into the ground and extend your legs back up to a slightly bent knee position. Be sure your hips are tucked under and knees remain flexed. Try eight repetitions.

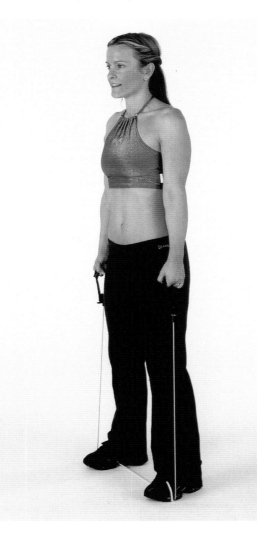

End position: Stand comfortably with an elongated spine. Look forward and keep your abdominal muscles relaxed.

Be aware: Throughout the exercise, you must keep your hips rolled under and chin tucked in.

It is often tempting to lift the chin toward the ceiling during the exercise. Resist this urge and keep your chin tucked in. Breathe as regularly as possible, inhaling on the way down and exhaling on the way up.

Alternative: You may shorten the length of the cord by doubling it, or you can pull your hands up higher.

Advanced: You may further increase the difficulty of this exercise by performing it with hand weights rather than a stretch cord.

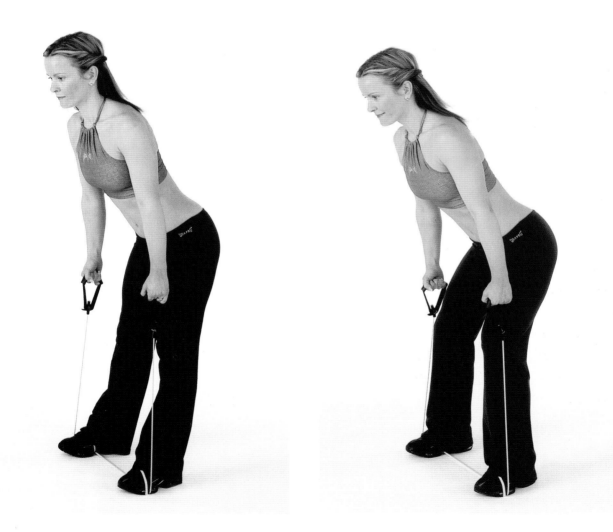

Balanced Leg Extension

Level: Beginner
Suitable for: Elite athletes
Unsuitable for: Seniors and pregnant women
Area of concentration: Psoas

For those of you who marvel at the balance, skill, and coordination of ice skaters or roller bladers, here is your chance to give skating a try without the cold ice or hard concrete. The Balanced Leg Extension can even be done on flat ground, which may be a good way for beginners to ease into the skill.

This is your chance to test your core strength and sense of balance. The Bosu ball is essentially a Swiss ball chopped in half and mounted upon a flat board, creating a non-stable yet not particularly threatening environment. The balance or core board is another de-stabilizing device that could also be used. It can be used for a variety of exercises, but is particularly good for testing your balance. This exercise offers you the opportunity to explore the full range of your hip joint, activating all the support muscles between your core and your legs.

Start position: Stand in front of the Bosu ball with your feet shoulder width apart and hands at your side. Roll your pelvis underneath so that your spine is long and extended. You should feel the stability of your entire foot pressing into the ground. Keep your abdomen relaxed. Focus your eyes forward and keep your chin level with the ground and tucked in so that it is not protruding. Imagine that your head is reaching up toward the ceiling.

Exercise: Continuing to fix your gaze forward, place your left foot on the crest (the top) of the Bosu ball, or balance board, and extend your relaxed arms forward for a counterbalance as you transfer your weight over your left leg and lift your right leg behind you. You might notice that this posture resembles an ice skater pushing off one blade and gliding. Be sure that you keep your hips rolled under and feel your entire foot against the top of the ball. Your armpits should press down in order to seat your shoulders. You will notice some instability from the inherent nature of the ball, but this activates your proprioception capabilities in your core and connective tissue. Hold this stance for 15 seconds, arms and right leg extended, then gradually return your right leg to the ground.

End position: Keeping your eyes focused forward, carefully transfer your weight from your left leg back to your right as you shift off of the Bosu ball. You will finally return to a standing position with your weight equally distributed on both feet. Repeat the exercise with your right leg bearing your weight on the ball and your left leg elevated. Try for longer durations.

Be aware: Remember to keep your spine elongated and your hip rolled under. You might be tempted to look down at your feet for a feeling of stability, but this creates the tendency to slump and defeats the purpose of the exercise. Continue breathing in a relaxed fashion, assuring that you do not hold your breath.

Intermediate: Using the same range of motion make it more difficult by lifting your knee.

Advanced: Using the same range of motion, lift your knee, then return it to a fully extended position.

Balanced Knee Lift

Level: Intermediate

Suitable for: Elite athletes

Unsuitable for: Seniors and pregnant women

Area of concentration: Iliopsoas, gluteal, erector spinae, and abdomen

From the basic skill of balancing with one leg extended, this is a more dynamic alternative. The exercise involves moving through a range of motion and maintaining balance on an unstable environment. This exercise can also be done on flat ground, which may be a good way for beginners to ease into the skill.

The Balanced Knee Lift offers you the opportunity to explore the full range of your hip joint, activating all the support muscles that attach your core to your legs. You might imagine yourself to be a high jumper, just ready to launch over the high bar.

Start position: Stand in front of the Bosu ball with your feet shoulder width apart and hands at your side. Roll your pelvis underneath so that your spine is long and extended. Feel the stability of your entire foot pressing into the ground and keep your abdomen relaxed. Keep your eyes focused forward and your chin level with the ground, tucked in and not protruding. Your head should reach toward the ceiling.

Exercise: Continuing to fix your gaze forward, place your left foot on the crest (the top) of the Bosu ball, or balance board, and extend your relaxed arms forward for a counterbalance as you transfer your weight over your left leg and lift your right leg behind you. Be sure that you keep your hips rolled under and feel your entire foot against the top of the ball. Your armpits press down in order to seat your shoulders. You will notice some instability from the inherent nature of the ball, but this activates your proprioceptive capabilities in your core and connective tissue. Now slowly lift your right knee to a relatively comfortable position in front of you, about hip high or more if you can retain your balance. Hold this stance for 15 seconds, arms closer to your body, then gradually return your right leg to the ground.

End position: Keeping your eyes focused forward, carefully transfer your weight from your left leg back to your right as you shift off the Bosu ball. Finally, return to a standing position with your weight equally distributed on both feet. Repeat the exercise with your right leg bearing your weight on the ball and your left leg elevated. Try for longer durations.

Be aware: Remember to keep your spine elongated and your hips rolled under. You might be tempted to look down at your feet for a feeling of stability, but this creates the tendency to slump the back and defeats the purpose of the exercise. Continue breathing in a relaxed fashion and do not hold your breath.

Intermediate/advanced: You could add ankle weights to both legs to challenge yourself further.

Advanced: Using the same range of motion, lift your knee, then return to a fully extended position.

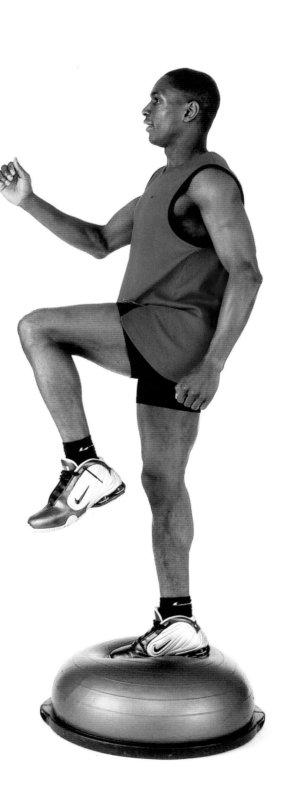

Swiss Ball

Swiss Kegels

Level: Beginner

Suitable for: All

Area of concentration: Pubococcygeal muscles

If you have worked your way through the book, then by now you may have begun to notice a pattern to the exercises you have undertaken. With each one, positioning of the trunk of the body is of primary importance to successfully completing the movement. Why should this be so? Why bother to be precise when, after all, we are only exercising?

The answer is targeting and isolation. As we target and strengthen areas that have been neglected over the years, we can rebuild and tone the areas that have become weakened. It takes special effort to keep our bodies fully toned and properly functioning, largely because the daily activities we experienced just a few short generations ago have primarily disappeared for many individuals. Our bodies don't have to work as much as they once did.

Because of these special toning needs, which require more than just routine exercises, we must improvise with special tools and techniques. One of these is the Swiss ball. The Swiss ball enables us to comfortably and precisely isolate areas of our core and exercise them within the context of the rest of our body. In some sense, the Swiss ball offers us a land-based version of suspension, similar to water. It removes hard ground stress points and requires that we coordinate the movements of muscles, tendons, and ligaments in unison.

This section explores the types of exercises you can do with the Swiss ball. By moving slowly, you can feel for and identify the elusive muscles deep inside, such as the psoas, that have such dramatic effect upon spinal stability and alignment. You can tune your proprioception just by sitting on the ball, because you are constantly shifting your foot pressure just to stabilize your seated position.

Swiss Kegels are a good place to start because you can establish your feeling of stability while working the pubococcygeal muscles of the pelvic floor.

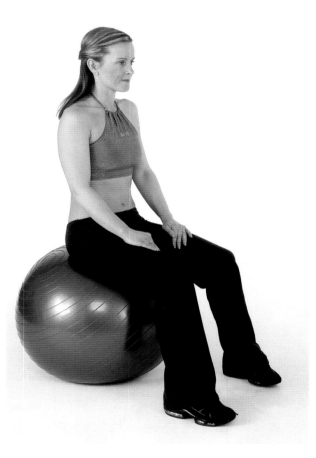

Start position: Take a seated position on a Swiss ball, bringing your upper leg roughly parallel with the ground and forming a 90-degree angle in your knees. If you feel a little uncertain about your stability, be sure that you experiment on a soft mat and consider using a wall or attached dancer's stretch bar for added stability on your side. Be wary of slipping off or rolling into the wall, of course. If you have a partner to help you, this may offer a better alternative. Never position a hard surface behind you.

Sit with your spine feeling elongated and your weight resting upon your sitting bones. Breathe in and out comfortably. Make sure there are no hard surfaces directly behind you; you have to protect your head.

Exercise: Feel the pubococcygeal muscles that connect your coccyx to your pubic bone directly beneath you as you sit on the ball. Squeeze them while relaxing your abdomen, hold for three seconds, then release. Repeat this eight times.

Feel your feet press into the ground to provide stability, and feel the connection of muscles working all the way up your legs to your core. You may press down into the ball and squeeze your buttocks if you feel unstable.

End position: Sit with your spine feeling elongated. Imagine your head as if it is lifting to the ceiling. Keep your eyes forward, your spine straight, and your lower spine sinking straight down into the ball.

Be aware: Be careful that you keep your spine elongated and your shoulders seated. You want your exercise effort to come from your core, so keep your chin tucked in. Breathe out as you contract and inhale as you release throughout the exercise, and press down from your armpits. Try to avoid bouncing on the ball and keep your movements smooth.

Intermediate: From a prone position, try doing hip thrusts with a leg squeeze.

Rotations

Level: Beginner

Suitable for: Everyone

Area of concentration: Pubococcygeal muscles, iliopsoas, erector spinae

After you have started with the basic Kegel exercise on the Swiss ball, you can try something more dynamic. By moving slowly, you will have the opportunity to feel for and identify the elusive muscles deep inside, such as the psoas, that have such dramatic effect upon our spinal stability and alignment. This exercise is a simple movement that everyone, including seniors and pregnant women, may enjoy.

Start position: Take a seated position on a Swiss ball, bringing your upper leg roughly parallel with the ground, and forming a 90-degree angle in your knees. Slightly lower is even better. If you feel a little uncertain about your stability, be sure that you experiment on a soft mat and consider using a wall or attached dancer's stretch bar for added stability. Be wary of slipping off or rolling into the wall, of course. If you have a partner to help you, this may offer a better alternative.

Sit with your spine feeling very elongated and your weight resting upon your sitting bones. Press down in your armpits. Breathe comfortably. Your arms may provide a stabilizing balance by positioning them away from your side with your palms facing downward. Alternatively, sit with your hands resting on your thighs. In this position, you are ready to protect yourself should you roll too far off the ball. Make sure there are no hard surfaces directly behind you; you must protect your head.

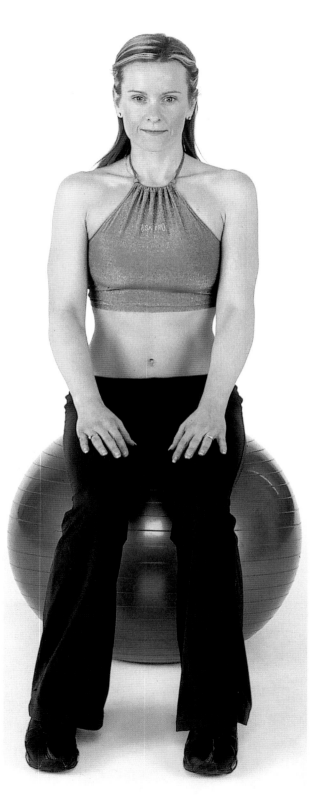

Exercise: Begin to roll your hips in a circular clockwise direction. This is an excellent opportunity to explore your range of motion and "open" your pelvis area, by relaxing your connective tissue and encouraging flexibility. Next try rolling your hips counterclockwise.

Feel your feet press into the ground for stability, and feel the connection of muscles working all the way up your legs to your core. You may press down into the ball to accommodate your rotating hips.

You may further explore range of motion by limiting your movements laterally (side to side) or longitudinally (front to back). Again, you are looking to relax and extend the connective tissue within the pelvis, without slumping out of a straight alignment.

End position: Sit with an elongated spine, facing forward.

Be aware: Be careful that you keep your spine elongated and your shoulders seated. You want your exercise effort to come from your core, so keep your chin tucked in. Breathe out as you contract and inhale as you release throughout the exercise, and press down from your armpits. Try to avoid bouncing on the ball and keep your movements smooth.

Intermediate/advanced: Raise your arms higher while performing the exercise

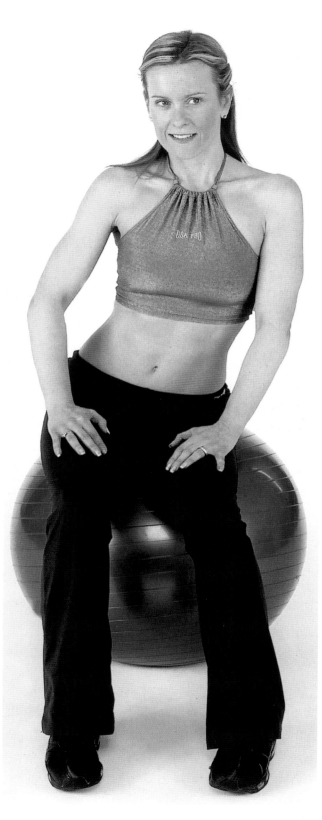

Contralateral Arm/Leg Extension

Level: Intermediate

Unsuitable for: Pregnant women

Area of Concentration: Erector spinae

Once you get a feeling for balancing on the Swiss ball, you may begin to try some prone and supine exercises that amplify those you already do on the mat. The Gluteal Crunch exercise, or "Superman," is one example where you can use a Swiss ball to get you off the hard mat and test your stability.

Start position: From the prone position, face down on the Swiss ball with your right arm stabilizing you against the ground. Extend the right leg straight back until you have formed one long line from your head, down your spine to your heel. Keep your hips tucked under to help maintain this straight line. Extend your left arm simultaneously to a position parallel with the ground and breathe from your abdomen.

Exercise: Continuing to fix your gaze at the ground, contract your gluteal and hamstring muscles while keeping your lower back relaxed and straight. Raise your leg as high as is comfortable, while simultaneously raising your left arm to a similar height. Allow them to lower to below parallel in a controlled manner. That is one repetition.

You may repeat the up and down motion for your desired number of repetitions, then change to a right arm/left leg combination.

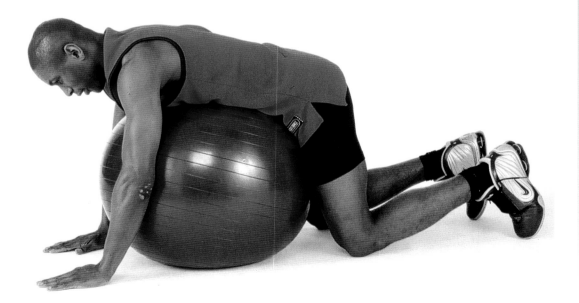

End position: Resume the prone position on the Swiss ball, breathing comfortably.

Be aware: Remember to keep your spine elongated and breathe out with each extension, back in with each lowering/relaxation.

Advanced: You may place weights around your ankles and wrist.

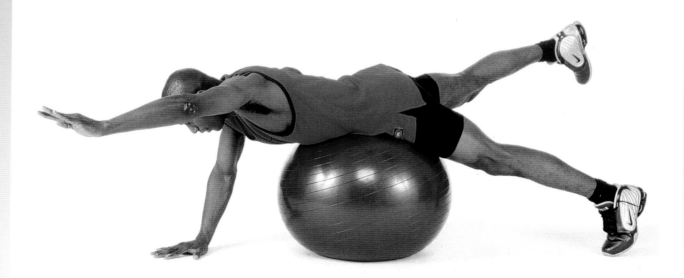

Full Range Crunch

Level: Intermediate
Suitable for: Healthy individuals
Unsuitable for: Pregnant women
Area of concentration: Abdomen, psoas, erector spinae

The Swiss ball crunch is a nice opportunity to experiment with your range of motion a bit. Try relaxing the normal discipline of keeping a long straight spine and tucked in hips in favor of using the Swiss ball's soft, forgiving curve to sense your lower spine's full range. You can experiment to the extent that the movement feels comfortable to you or apply the normal crunch discipline of a straight spine.

A gentle hyperextension of the lower spine does give you a feeling of the muscles necessary to roll your pelvis back under and create the tuck. Against the bouncy ball and without the strain of a hard floor, the abdominals may enjoy a gentle elongation and stretch.

Start position: The Full Range Crunch can be completed with or without wall anchoring. Without anchoring, you simply place your feet flat on the ground while sitting on the Swiss ball, knees at 90 degrees, and sink your lower back into the curvature of the ball. Relax your arms and hands over your chest. Breathe in and out comfortably.

Exercise: Arch your lower back into the contour of the ball gently, and allow the rest of your spine to follow this arch. Next, contract your abdomen muscles and

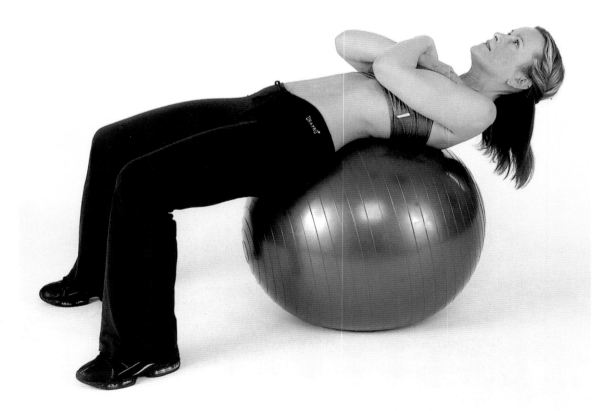

roll your hips under, creating a feeling of contraction from both your pelvis area and your lower abdomen.

Be careful not to pull with your upper neck muscles or bounce off the ball to attain your crunch movement. Lift your chest with your contraction. The whole point of the exercise is to work the lower core muscles and explore the full range of motion.

Hold that contraction for two seconds and squeeze your muscles. Lower yourself slowly back to the curvature of the ball. Repeat this motion eight times.

End position: Lie against the ball with an elongated spine and abdominal muscles relaxed.

Be aware: It is often tempting to lift the chin toward the ceiling during the exercise. Resist this urge and only lift your shoulder blades as high as you can by using your abdominal muscles. Breathe as regularly as possible throughout the exercise. Each contraction of the abdomen muscles should correspond with an exhalation, while each relaxation should correspond with inhalation.

Intermediate/advanced: You may perform this exercise with a free weight, securely fastened, on your chest.

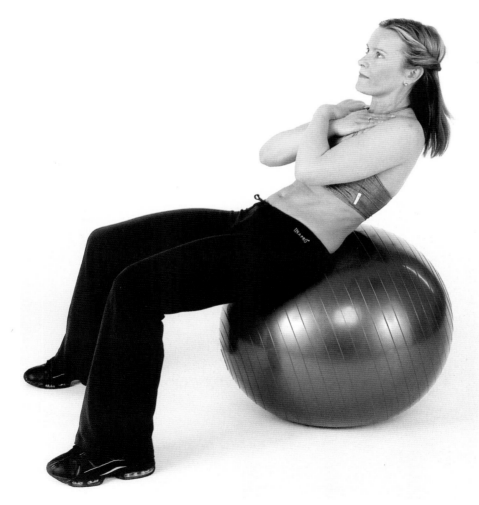

Butterfly or Back Crunch

Level: Intermediate

Suitable for: Healthy individuals

Unsuitable for: Pregnant women

Area of concentration: Erector spinalis, upper back

Back crunches may be performed on a mat, on a table with a partner holding your legs, on a Roman chair, or on a Swiss ball. The Swiss ball, especially, is a rather effective and forgiving method of exploring your full range of motion, using your erector spinalis muscles while elongating your abdominals.

Start position: From the prone position, face down on the Swiss ball with your hips pressing into it. Anchor your feet against a wall by bending your knees slightly and pressing your feet into the low corner of the wall where it meets the floor. Place your hands along the side of your neck lightly. Feel the balls of your feet dig into the ground, gripping it so that you have a stable yet flexible and bouncy platform from which to extend up. Roll your hips into the ball, feeling pressure on your pubic bone as you straighten your spine.

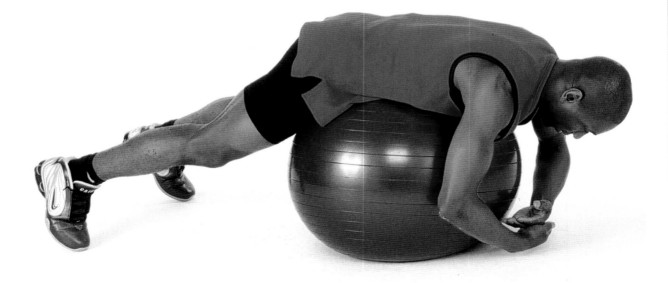

Exercise: Breathe out as you contract the lower back and gluteal muscles and raise your upper body. Hold the upright position for three seconds, then slowly lower yourself back down around the ball.

You may add an oblique twist to this basic lumbar crunch. Just twist to each side after your basic crunch, keeping your hands in position.

End position: Return to a relaxed prone position and allow the curvature of the ball to induce some stretching of the upper (thoracic) vertebrae.

Be aware: Remember to keep your spine elongated. Breathe out with each extension and back in with each lowering/relaxation.

Intermediate/advanced: You may place weights around your wrists.

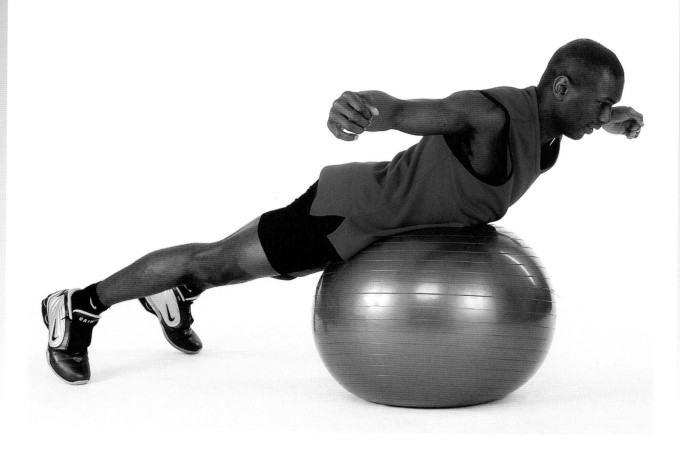

Leg Raises

Level: Intermediate

Suitable for: Healthy individuals

Unsuitable for: Pregnant women

Area of concentration: Erector spinalis, glutes, psoas elongation

Leg raises can also be performed while holding onto the end of a padded exercise table. Normally, your legs would hang off the end and you would raise and lower them. Swiss ball offers a chance to do this exercise far more comfortably. To avoid sore hips and stiff tables, it is worth giving this method a try. Using a Swiss ball is a rather effective and forgiving method of exploring this full range of motion, using your erector spinalis, glutes and elongating your psoas.

Start position: From the prone position, face down on the Swiss ball with your hips pressing into it. Place your hands on the ground as a steadying anchor. Roll your hips into the ball, feeling pressure on your pubic bone as you straighten your spine. Your body should be just about horizontal, and your upper body should stay horizontal throughout the exercise.

Exercise: Breathe out as you contract the lower back and gluteal muscles and raise your legs together. Hold the upright position for three seconds, then slowly

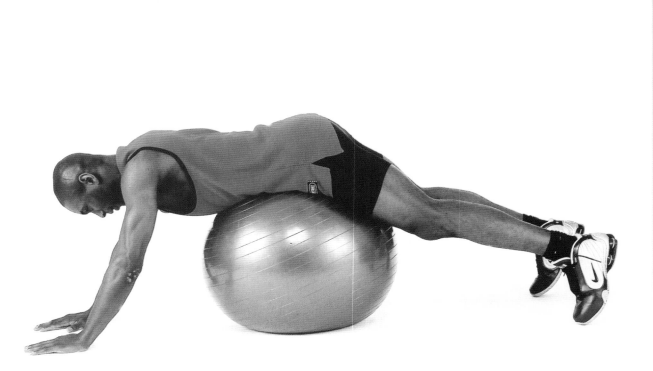

lower your legs back down. Use your hips to press into the ball as a fulcrum.

You may also try one leg at a time, which is slightly more forgiving if you feel some discomfort around your lower back.

End position: Return to a relaxed prone position and allow the curvature of the ball to induce some stretching of the upper (thoracic) vertebrae.

Be aware: Remember to keep your spine elongated. Breathe out with each extension, back in with each lowering/relaxation.

Intermediate/advanced: You may place weights around your ankles.

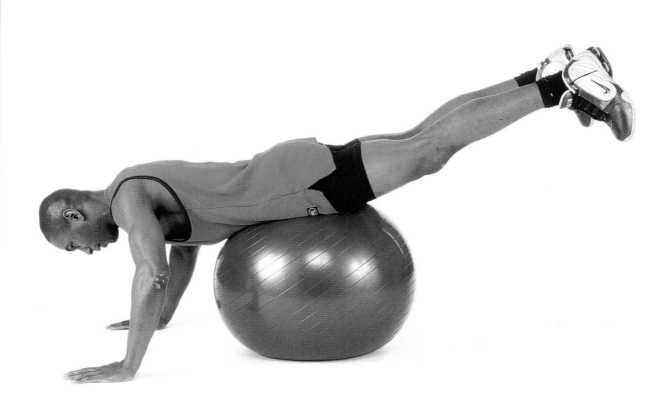

Weights

The Free Weight Crunch Exercise

Level: Intermediate/advanced

Suitable for: Healthy individuals, elite athletes

Unsuitable for: Prenatal

Area of concentration: Abdomen

If you are serious about core training, then to increase the difficulty you can add weights to your basic exercises. The simplest and most direct method for adding weight is to secure plate-style free weights directly on the chest. All the disciplines of the standard crunch apply. In this exercise, you can use your hands to hold the weight on your chest. You may also use small dumbbell style weights, but they should also be positioned over the chest.

Start position: Lie on the floor or a mat, facing the ceiling, with your spine comfortably relaxed and touching the floor along its entire length. With your feet flat on the ground and shoulder width apart, flex your knees to a right-angle position.

Roll your hips under to elongate your lower spine. Hold a relatively light free weight to your chest with your palms facing downward right below your neck. Breathe in and out comfortably.

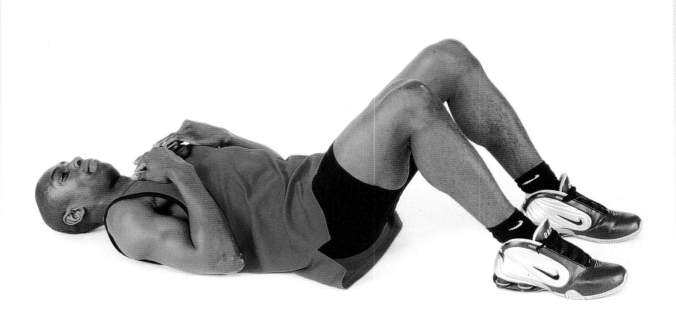

Exercise: Contract your abdomen muscles until you lift your shoulder blades off the ground. Keep your lower back flat and do not lift it off the mat. Concentrate on thrusting your chest toward the ceiling, while keeping your chin tucked in.

Hold at the top of the movement for two seconds and squeeze your muscles. Lower yourself slowly back to the mat. Repeat this motion eight times.

End position: Lie flat with an elongated spine and your abdominal muscles relaxed.

Be aware: It is often tempting to lift the chin toward the ceiling during this exercise. Resist this urge and only lift your shoulder blades as high as you can by using your abdominal muscles. Breathe as regularly as possible throughout the exercise. Each contraction of the abdomen muscles should correspond with an exhalation, while each relaxation should correspond with inhalation.

Advanced: You may perform this exercise on an incline bench with a free weight resting on your upper chest, or in standing position using a stretch cord or machine weights.

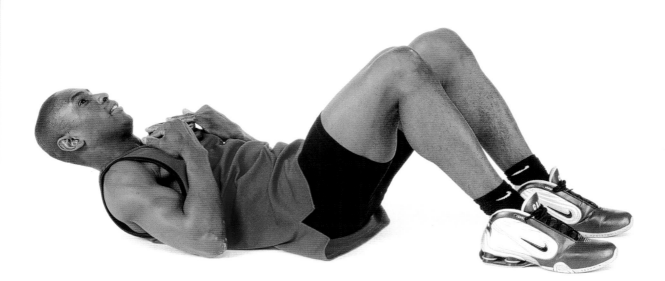

Oblique Crunch or Side Crunch

█ Level: Intermediate/advanced
█ Suitable for: Elite athletes
█ Area of Concentration: Obliques

The use of free weights creates a more dynamic exercise for the oblique muscle system, as well as an opportunity to test your core balance. This is a core body exercise that involves the whole body. Maintain a correct posture to protect your back.

Start position: Stand with your feet about shoulder width apart, and weights on either side of your feet. Your hips should be rolled under, knees slightly bent, shoulders down, and heels pressing into the ground.

Pick up the weights without slumping your spine. Keep your eyes forward and your chin tucked in. Stand straight up, knees slightly bent.

Exercise: Begin by contracting the oblique muscles on your right hand side and allowing the obliques on your left hand side to extend. Be sure your hips are tucked

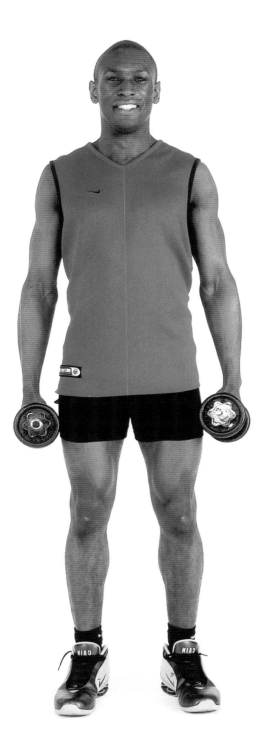

under and your knees remain flexed. Hold that side crunch for three seconds, then return to standing straight and stop for one second. Repeat for the opposite side. Aim for eight repetitions for each side.

End position: Stand with an elongated spine. Look forward with your abdominal muscles relaxed.

Be aware: Throughout the exercise, you must keep your hips rolled under and chin tucked in. Breathe as regularly as possible throughout the exercise.

Advanced: You may increase the difficulty of this exercise by adding heavier weights.

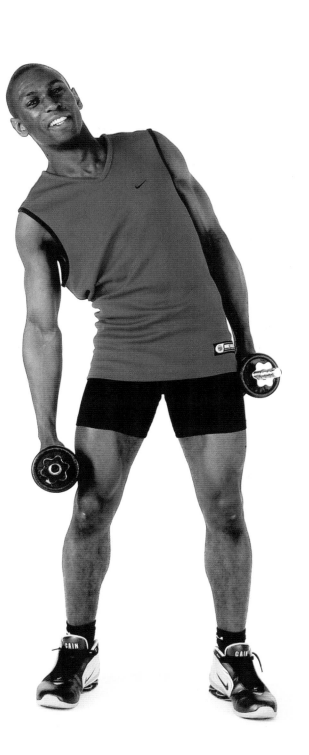

Dead Lift

Level: Advanced

Suitable for: Elite athletes

Unsuitable for: Seniors, back injury, pregnant women

Area of Concentration: Iliopsoas

The free weight dead lift is traditionally a mark of true athleticism, where only the well-informed and well-conditioned dare tread. Improper alignment or sloppy execution has been a source of injury for many practicing weight lifters. However, for the healthy individual, there is absolutely no reason not to try dead lifts. The key is proper alignment combined with relatively light hand weights.

Start position: Stand with your feet about shoulder width apart, and weights on either side of your feet. Your hips should be rolled under, knees slightly bent, shoulders down, and heels pressing into the ground.

Pick up the weights without slumping your spine. Keep your eyes forward, and your chin tucked in.

You may vary this exercise by keeping your legs straight, but be very careful not to strain your lower spine and ligaments.

Exercise: Bend from your hip joints, certain that your knees do not extend forward further than the vertical line rising straight up from your toes. You should experience a flexing sensation at the point where your leg joins your core body. Be sure to keep your hips rolled under and do not allow your lower spine to arch.

Next, slowly press your heels into the ground and extend your legs back up to a slightly bent knee

position. Be sure your hips are tucked under and knees remain flexed. Try eight repetitions.

End position: Stand comfortably with an elongated spine. Look forward keeping your abdominal muscles relaxed.

Be aware: Throughout the exercise, you must keep your hips rolled under and chin tucked in. It is often tempting to lift the chin toward the ceiling during the exercise. Resist this urge and keep your chin tucked in. Breathe regularly.

Advanced: You may increase the free weight resistance and technical difficulty by switching to mounted barbell free weights.

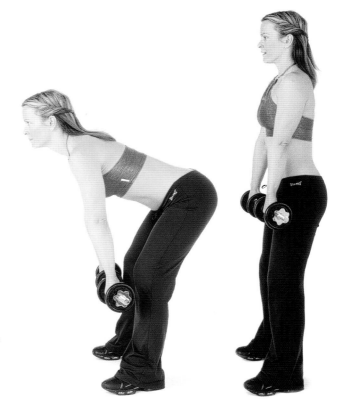

Free Weight Lunge

Level: Intermediate/advanced
Suitable for: Healthy individuals/elite athletes
Unsuitable for: Seniors, back injury, pregnant
women

The lunge exercise may at first seem to be aimed at leg strength development. In fact, the lunge works the iliopsoas and gluteal muscle groups in addition to exercising the hamstring.

Start position: Stand with your feet about shoulder width apart, and weights on either side of your feet. Your hips should be rolled under, knees slightly bent, shoulders down, and heels pressing into the ground.

Pick up the weights without slumping your spine. Keep your eyes forward and your chin tucked in.

Exercise: With your right foot, make a step forward that feels slightly longer than normal, yet not uncomfortable. As you gain confidence, you may step further. Allow your right leg to lower you slowly down until your upper thigh is parallel to the ground. Sink only as low as is comfortable. Roll up onto your toes on your back foot, the left, to allow this lunge step. Your left knee will probably tap the ground.

Now push back up with your right foot, as you keep your hip tucked under, and feel the core muscles working for you. Raise yourself up and step back to your standing position, then repeat with the left leg leading into the lunge. Try eight on each leg.

End position: Stand comfortably with an elongated spine, feet shoulder width apart. Gaze forward with your abdominal muscles relaxed.

Be aware: For stability, be sure that you feel your weight pressing into your heel on the lunging foot. Keep your spine long and your torso relatively straight up and down during the lunge. Throughout the exercise, you must keep your hips rolled under and chin tucked in. Breathe as regularly as possible throughout the exercise. Try inhaling on the lunge and exhaling on the way up.

Alternative/advanced: You may increase the free weight resistance and combine the lunge with a step platform.

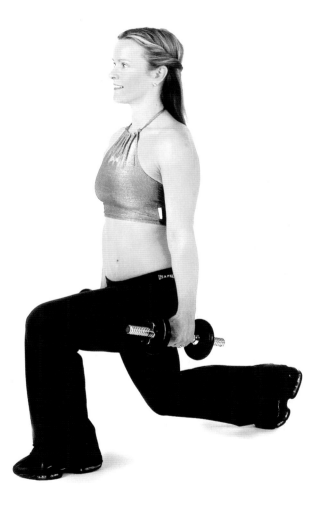

Hip Extension

Level: Advanced

Suitable for: All

Area of concentration: Erector spinalis, gluteals

Hip extensions are first learned on the mat or Swiss ball. Using a stacked weight and cable system or a targeted machine, you can make the basic exercise that much more challenging. If you have trouble with the weights, go back to the freestanding exercise or try performing it in water.

Start position: Stand in front of the stacked weight system, with the pulley at the bottom position. Place the connection strap on the right ankle and steady yourself by holding the frame or handle of the machine with your left hand.

Your hips should be rolled under, knees slightly bent, shoulders down, and heels pressing into the ground.

Exercise: With your left leg slightly bent, extend your right leg and hip backward. Repeat eight times and then do the same for the left leg. Move slowly to resist bouncing.

End position: Stand comfortably with an elongated spine, feet shoulder width apart. Look forward with your abdominal muscles relaxed.

Be aware: For stability, be sure that you feel your weight pressing into your heel on the standing leg. Keep your spine elongated and your torso relatively straight up and down during the sweep as you feel your abdominals stretch. Throughout the exercise, you must keep your hips rolled under and your chin tucked in. Breathe as regularly as possible.

Alternative: You may perform this in water.

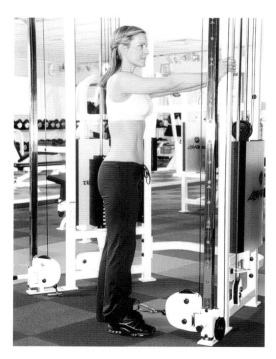 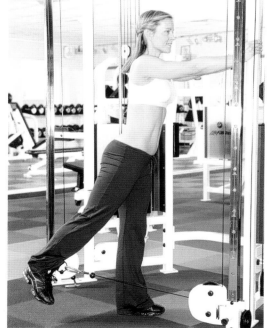

Adduction/Abduction

Level: Beginner

Suitable for: All

Area of concentration: Iliopsoas, gluteals, adductors

Using a stacked weight and cable system or a targeted machine, you can make the basic adduction/abduction exercise that much more challenging.

Start position: Stand sideways to the stacked weight and pulley machine, left leg closest, with the pulley at the bottom position. Place the connection strap on the right ankle and steady yourself by holding the frame of the machine with your left hand. Alternatively, place the strap on the ankle closest to the machine.

Exercise: With your standing leg slightly bent, make a sweeping motion with the other leg across the front of your body and back. Repeat eight times for both legs.

End position: Stand comfortably with an elongated spine, feet shoulder width apart. Look forward with your abdominal muscles relaxed.

Be aware: For stability, be sure that you press your weight into the heel of your standing leg. Keep your spine elongated and your torso relatively straight. Keep your hips rolled under and chin tucked in. Breathe regularly.

Alternative: You may perform this in water.

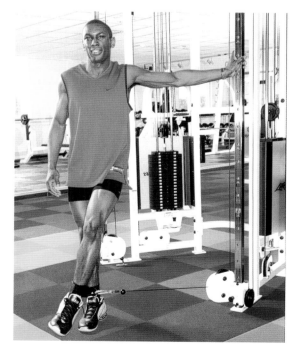
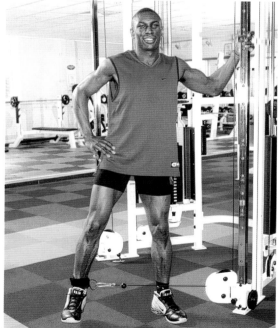

Standing Pull Down Crunch

Level: Advanced

Suitable for: Elite athletes, healthy individuals

Unsuitable for: Pregnant women

Area of concentration: Abdomen

The Standing Pull Down Crunch can be effectively completed using the stacked, pulley-based weight set available in any gym. This exercise is an alternative to simply performing a crunch on the floor with a weight plate mounted upon the chest. The added effect of standing while performing the exercise may also lend an aspect of balance and tone to the core. In general, the Standing Crunch exercise, whether with cord or stacked pulley weights, can be viewed as an alternative geared to the elite athlete looking for added challenge.

One advantage of the stacked weight system is the ability to easily choose your resistance level and move up gradually as your strength and skill level dictates. Whether you perform this exercise in the seated, kneeling or standing position, be careful not to strain the lower spine by allowing it to curve or hyperextend.

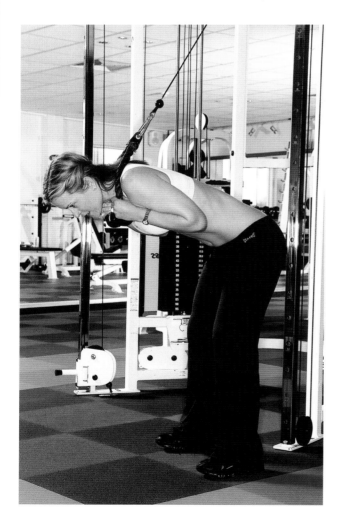

Start position: Stand underneath the suspended pulley associated with a stacked weight system. Your feet should be about shoulder width apart, legs straight. Your hips should be rolled under, shoulders down, and heels pressing into the ground. Grasp the horizontal bar above your shoulders with the hand contact point near your shoulders as you bend 90 degrees at your hip joint (pelvic fold) and prepare to use your abdomen muscles. You may use a rope or towel wrapped around a fixed clasp as well.

Exercise: Contract your abdomen muscles only in order to pull down the stretch cord. By keeping your legs straight, you will experience a stretching in your hamstrings. You may also bend your knees slightly, but keep the discipline of a straight back and be sure to use only your abdominals for your range of motion.

End position: Bend 90 degrees at your hip, keeping your spine straight. Breathe comfortably.

Be aware: You are working only the upper abs in this exercise, so breathe out upon contraction and inhale upon release.

Alternative/advanced: Add more weight on the stack.

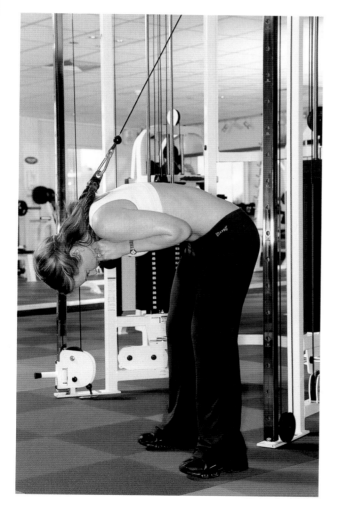

Seated Dead Lift

Level: Intermediate

Suitable for: Healthy individuals/athletes

Area of concentration: Lower spine, psoas

There is a clever way to simulate the first movement of the Dead Lift if you are a little intimidated by using a free weight lift. The trick is to sit down and use the stacked weight machine to isolate the lower back.

One advantage of the stacked weight system is the ability to easily choose your resistance level and move up gradually as your strength and skill level dictates.

Be careful not to strain your lower spine by allowing it to curve or hyperextend.

Start position: Sit in front of the row pulley associated with a stacked weight system. Your feet should be about shoulder width apart, your knees bent, and feet pressing against the frame of the weight machine. Your hips should be rolled under, shoulders down. Grasp the horizontal bar and hold it low with your arms straight.

You may vary this exercise by keeping your legs straight, but be very careful not to strain your lower spine and ligaments.

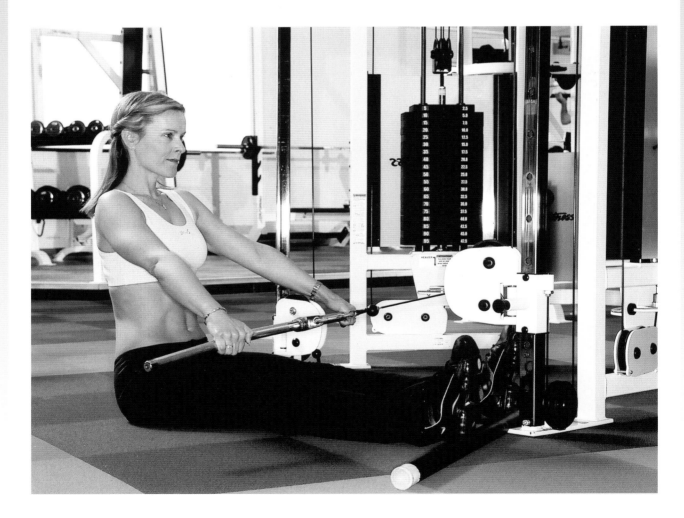

Exercise: Contract your abdomen muscles only in order to pull the row handle back. Move slowly back from about 90 degrees to 45 degrees, then slowly return to an upright position. Repeat eight times.

End position: Bend 90 degrees at your hip, spine straight. Breathe comfortably.

Be aware: Breathe out upon contraction and inhale upon release.

Advanced: Add more weight to the stack.

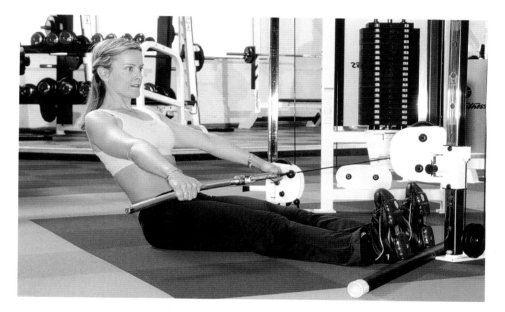

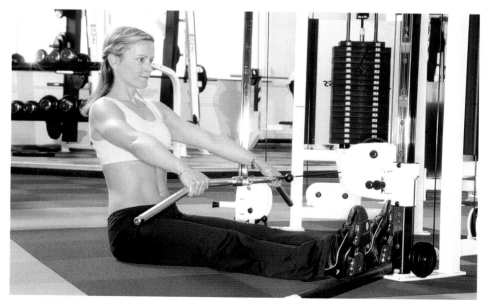

Trunk Rotation

Level: Advanced

Suitable for: All

Area of concentration: Erector spinalis, obliques, transverse abdominals

Weighted resistance exercises use the erector spinalis muscles as well as the obliques and transverse abdominis. Using a stacked weight and cable system or a targeted machine, you can work the core muscles within a contained range of motion as long as you are careful with alignment.

Start position: Stand with your left side facing the stacked weight system, with the pulley at the middle position. Hold the connection handle in your right hand and steady yourself by standing with your knees slightly flexed and feet shoulder width or a little further apart. Stand so that the weight is engaged when you place your right hand holding the handle on your right hip. You may keep your hand slightly away from your hip in a fixed position.

Your hips should be rolled under, shoulders pressing down, and heels pressing into the ground.

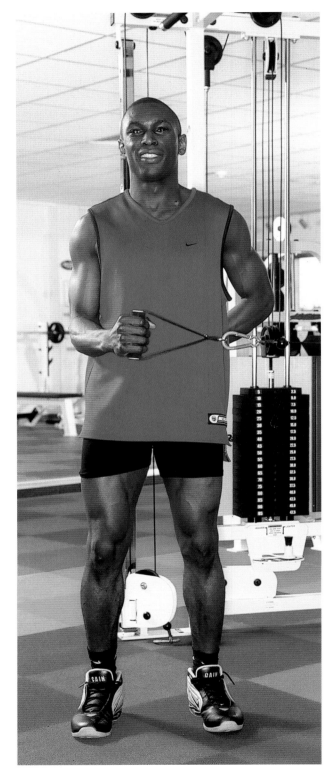

Exercise: Breathe out, turn your trunk to the right side, feeling pressure against your left leg. Slowly allow the weight resistance to turn you all the way back, completing one rotation. Try this eight times then switch position to your other side.

End position: Stand comfortably with an elongated spine, feet shoulder width apart. Look forward with your abdominal muscles relaxed.

Be aware: For stability, be sure that you feel your weight pressing into your heel on the pushing leg. Keep your spine elongated and your torso relatively straight up and down during the rotation as you feel your abdominals stretch. Throughout the exercise, you must keep your hips rolled under and chin tucked in. Breathe out on contraction and in on return.

Alternative: You may perform this with hand cords.

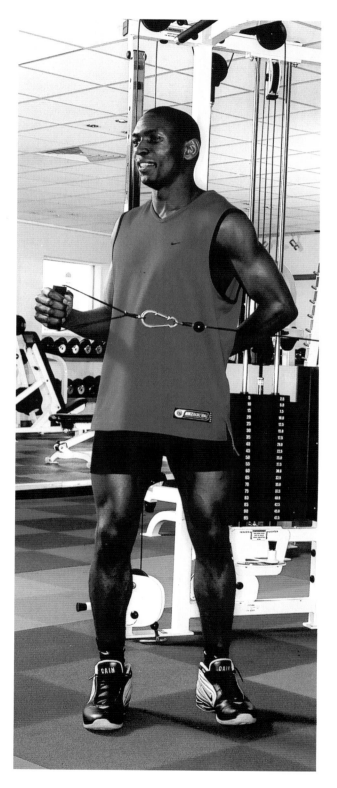

Trunk Rotation With High Anchor

Level: Advanced

Suitable for: All

Area of concentration: Erector spinalis, obliques, transverse abdominals

Once you have tried standard trunk rotation with a waist-high anchor, you may undertake a more dynamic trunk extension exercise. Using a stacked weight and cable system or stretchable cord, you can work the core muscles within a contained range of motion as long as you are careful with alignment.

Start position: Stand with your left side facing the stacked weight system, with the pulley at the upper position. Hold the connection handle in your right hand and steady yourself by standing with your knees slightly flexed and your feet shoulder width or a little further apart. Stand so that the weight is engaged when you place your right hand holding the handle on your right hip. You may keep your hand away from your hip in a fixed position to allow the cable to move across your chest.

Your hips should be rolled under, shoulders pressing down, and heels pressing into the ground.

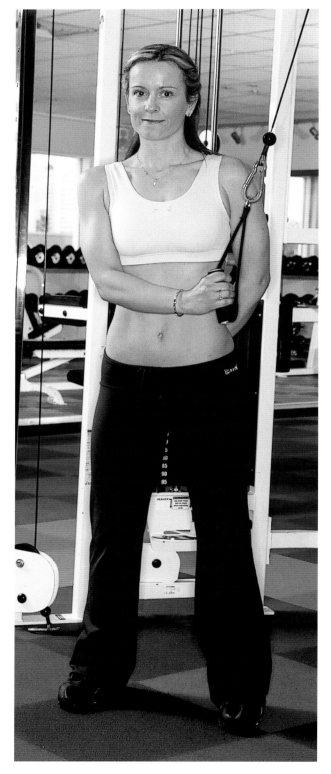

Exercise: Breathe out, turn your trunk to the right side and pull down toward the floor off to your right, feeling pressure against your left leg. You are creating a diagonal movement against resistance. Slowly allow the weight resistance to turn you all the way back, completing one rotation. Try this eight times then switch position to your other side.

End position: Stand comfortably with an elongated spine, feet shoulder width apart. Look forward with your abdominal muscles relaxed.

Be aware: For stability, be sure that you feel your weight pressing into your heel on the pushing leg. Keep your spine elongated and your torso relatively straight during the rotation as you feel your abdominals stretch. Throughout the exercise, you must keep your hips rolled under and your chin tucked in. Start with light weights and be careful of your lower spine. Breathe out on contraction and in on return.

Alternative: You may perform this with hand cords.

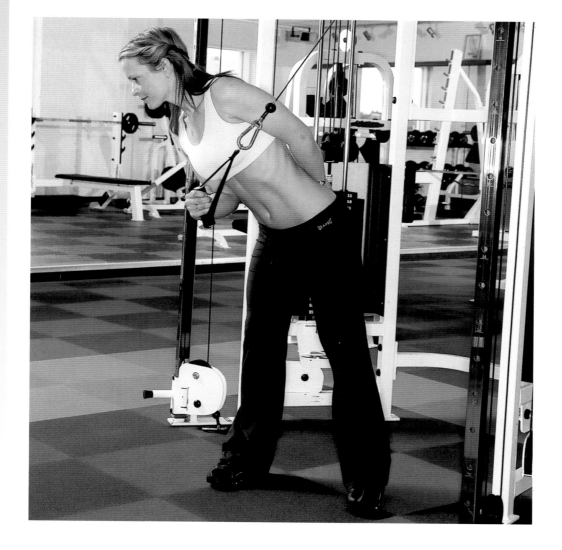

Trunk Rotation With Low Anchor

Level: Advanced

Suitable for: All

Area of concentration: Erector spinalis, obliques, transverse abdominals

Once you have tried a standard trunk rotation with a waist high anchor, you may undertake a more dynamic trunk extension exercise. Using a stacked weight and cable system or stretchable cord, you can work the core muscles within a contained range of motion as long as you are careful with alignment.

Start position: Stand with your left side facing the stacked weight system, with the pulley at the lower position. Hold the connection handle in your right hand and steady yourself by standing with your knees slightly flexed and feet shoulder width or a little further apart. Stand so that the weight is engaged when you place your right hand, holding the handle, on your right shoulder. You may hold your hand away from your body in a fixed position.

Your hips should be rolled under, shoulders pressing down, and heels pressing into the ground.

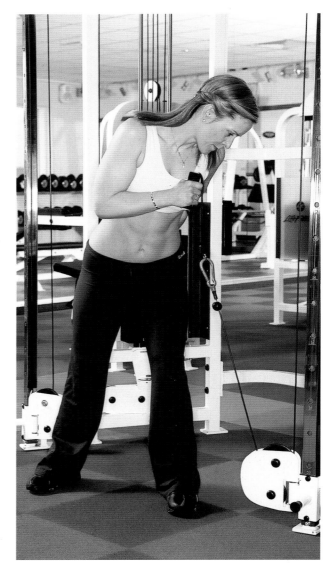

Exercise: Breathe out, turn your trunk to the right side and pull up toward the ceiling off to your right, feeling pressure against your left leg. Create a diagonal movement against resistance. Slowly allow the weight resistance to turn you all the way back, completing one rotation. Try this eight times then switch position to your other side.

End position: Stand comfortably with an elongated spine, feet shoulder width apart. Look forward with your abdominal muscles relaxed.

Be aware: For stability, be sure that you feel your weight pressing into your heel on the pushing leg. Keep your spine elongated and your torso relatively straight during the rotation as you feel your abdominals stretch. Throughout the exercise, you must keep your hips rolled under and chin tucked in. Start with light weights and be careful of your lower spine. Breathe out on contraction and in on return.

Alternative: You may perform this with hand cords.

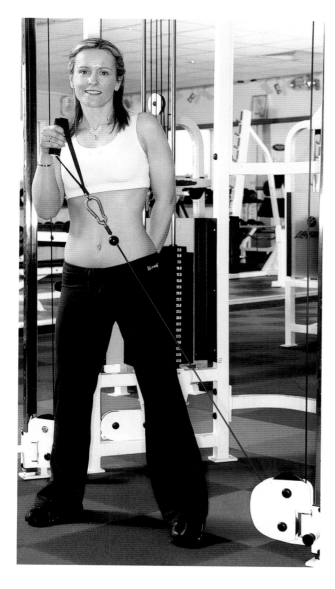

Gym Equipment

Crunch

Level: Beginner
Suitable for: Healthy individuals, elite athletes
Unsuitable for: Pregnant women
Area of concentration: Abdomen, iliopsoas

In addition to the specialized machines found in gyms around the globe, there are a seemingly infinite variety of "ab workout" devices. At first glance, any machine or device that you enjoy using and will continue to use has some value. In order to determine physiological merit, however, ask yourself if the machine forces you to curve your spine unnaturally or prohibits you from keeping an elongated spine.

With any machine found in a gym, try one repetition at a very light weight. This way you may test your range of motion and determine your comfort level. Gym machines tend to have a stacked set of plate weights; a set of padded lever arms that connect to a fulcrum shaped interface and transmit the work accomplished by your body to move the weight.

Resistance can also be provided by compressed air cylinders, cords, bands, metal strips, almost anything you can think of that is hard to move, lift, bend or compress. There are gluteal and hamstring machines, hip flexors, crunch and fly extensions. Always be careful to sit squarely in the chair and watch for vulnerable joints, such as the knee, when pressing against an ankle pad. The best advice is to seek the help of a personal trainer in assuring that you are using the machine or device correctly.

The incline bench is an easily recognizable piece of equipment meant to provide some variability to resistance training. One end provides an "anchor," a place where you may secure a foothold or handhold that prevents you from sliding down the incline. The other end is open and the angle of inclination is adjustable.

The basic incline crunch involves exactly the same hand and body positioning and behavior as a crunch performed on the floor, along with the same exercise disciplines. The angle of inclination provides resistance, and you might feel a slight increase of blood pressure, a "rush of blood to the head," as you anchor your feet in the high position. Start with a relatively low angle of inclination. By slowly returning to the bench, you are performing a decline crunch. You can work the abdominals both ways.

Start position: Secure your feet according to the type of anchor on the bench. Most provide padded rollers, under which you slip your feet as your knees slip over another higher padded roller. Be careful not to strain your cruciate ligaments in your knees while performing any motions on the incline bench. The effort must come from the targeted area.

Roll your hips under to elongate your lower spine. Relax your arms and hands on your chest with your palms facing downward right below your neck. Breathe in and out comfortably.

Exercise: Contract your abdomen muscles until you lift your shoulder blades off the incline bench. Your lower back stays flat and you do not need to lift it off the bench. Concentrate to thrust your chest toward the ceiling, while your chin stays tucked.

Hold at the top of the movement for two seconds and squeeze your muscles. Lower yourself slowly back to the mat. Repeat this motion eight times.

If you are feeling adventurous, try the full sit-up. Initiate the contraction in the same way that you did the crunch, but continue the motion until your chest is close to your knees. Remember to breathe out all the way up, then hold that position, then slowly inhale while lowering yourself back to the bench.

End position: Lie flat with an elongated spine and your abdominal muscles relaxed.

Be aware: It is often tempting to lift the chin toward the ceiling during the exercise. Resist this urge and only lift using your abdominal muscles. Breathe as regularly as possible throughout the exercise. Each contraction of the abdominal muscles should correspond with an exhalation, while each return to the bench should correspond with inhalation.

Advanced: You may perform this exercise with a free weight resting on your upper chest.

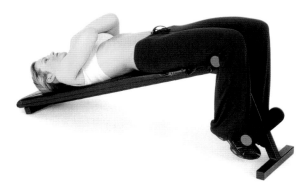
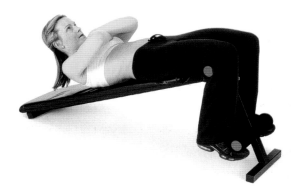

Crunch

Level: Intermediate

Suitable for: Healthy individuals, athletes

Unsuitable for: Pregnant women

Areas of concentration: Abdominals, psoas

Once you have determined your comfort zone for basic crunches and/or sit-ups on the incline board, you may want to add some extra resistance. Obviously, the quickest way to do so is to secure a free weight plate on your body and follow the same range of motion as the incline crunch.

The same disciplines apply in terms of hand position, spinal alignment, and the use of your abdominals in order to avoid neck strain.

Start position: Secure your feet according to the type of anchor on the bench. Most provide padded rollers under which you slip your feet as your knees slip over another higher padded roller. Be careful not to strain your cruciate ligaments in your knees while performing any motions on the incline bench. The effort must come from the targeted area.

Roll your hips under to elongate your lower spine. Hold the weight plate securely on your chest, and breathe in and out comfortably.

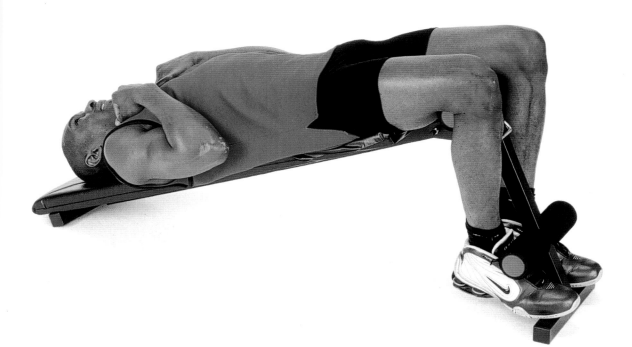

Exercise: Contract your abdomen muscles until you lift your shoulder blades off the incline bench. Keep your lower back flat and do not lift it off the bench. Concentrate on thrusting your chest toward the ceiling while your chin stays tucked in.

Hold at the top of the movement for two seconds and squeeze your muscles. Lower yourself slowly back to the bench. Repeat this motion eight times.

If you are feeling adventurous, try the full sit-up. Initiate the contraction in the same way that you did the crunch, but continue the motion until your chest is close to your knees. Remember to breathe out all the way up, then hold that position. Slowly inhale while lowering yourself back to the bench.

End position: Lie flat with an elongated spine and your abdominal muscles relaxed.

Be aware: It is often tempting to lift the chin toward the ceiling during the exercise. Resist this urge and only lift using your abdominal muscles. Breathe as regularly as possible throughout the exercise. Each contraction of the abdominal muscles should correspond with an exhalation, while each return to the bench should correspond with an inhalation.

Advanced: You may perform this exercise with a partner pressing on your shoulders in the direction opposite to your motion.

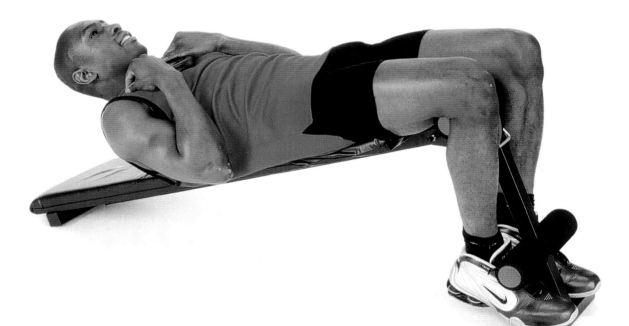

Roll Up and Jackknife

■ Level: Intermediate/advanced
■ Suitable for: Healthy individuals, elite athletes
■ Unsuitable for: Pregnant women
■ Area of concentration: Abdominals, erector spinae

The incline bench may be used for heads up as well as feet first exercises. Rather than anchor your ankles, try hanging on with both hands for another version of these types of exercises.

Start position: Lie back on the bench at no more than a 45-degree angle and hang on with both hands over your head. Make sure you feel your whole spine, from your neck all the way down to your lower vertebrae, touching the incline bench.

Roll your hips under to elongate your lower spine. Flex your hips at the fold and bring your bent knees all the way up to your chest.

Exercise: Contract your abdomen muscles until you lift your knees towards your shoulders. Hold at the top of the movement for two seconds and squeeze your muscles. Lower yourself slowly back to the bench. Repeat this motion eight times.

If you are feeling adventurous, try a jackknife. Initiate the contraction in the same way that you did the crunch, but this time keep your legs straight and

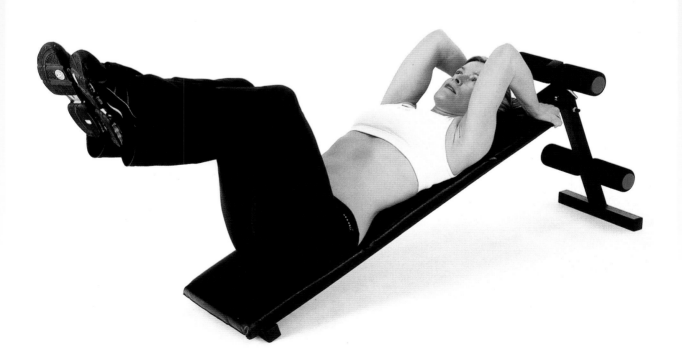

make sure your lower spine is flat to the bench. Be careful with this one; hyperextension is possible and this may cause strain. Use your own judgment. Remember to breathe out all the way up, then hold that position with your legs toward the ceiling. Slowly inhale while lowering yourself back to the bench.

End position: Lie flat with an elongated spine and your abdominal muscles relaxed.

Be aware: Only lift using your abdominal muscles. Breathe as regularly as possible throughout the exercise. Each contraction of the abdominal muscles should correspond with an exhalation, while each return to the bench should correspond with an inhalation.

Advanced: The advanced form of this exercise can be done vertically from a suspension rack.

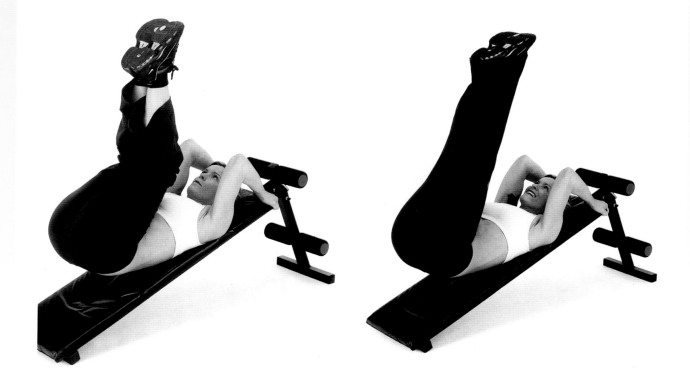

Leg Raise

Level: Beginner

Suitable for: Young people, elite athletes

Area of concentration: Iliopsoas, gluteals, pubococcygeals

In the free weight area of many gyms, you might find a suspensory rack. This device elevates and supports you through two padded arm rests and a padded back support. One nice feature of the rack is the lengthening effect you may experience on your iliopsoas and connective tissue in general.

There is a variety of core exercises you may perform from this platform, but it pays to be cautious. You are, after all, supporting your entire body weight upon both forearms, which can create unnatural strain in your shoulders. If you do feel stress in your rotator cuff or shoulders in general, there are plenty of mat-based alternatives available. In the absence of a suspensory rack, you may use a hanging bar to improvise the situation where your legs hang freely.

Start position: Mount the suspensory rack by resting both forearms on the pads and pressing gently with your lower spine against the padded back support. Your spine should be extended as straight as possible as your legs hang freely and feet are together.

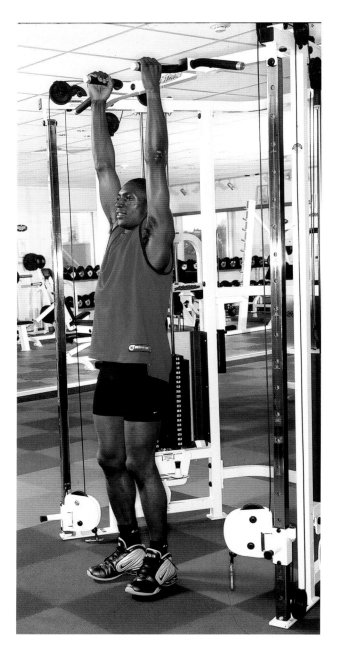

Exercise: Bend from your hip joints as you lift your knees toward your chest. You should experience a flexing sensation at the point where your leg joins your core body. Be sure to keep your hips rolled under and do not allow your lower spine to arch. Hold that position, then slowly release the legs back to the straight-down position. While completing the repetition, remember also to contract your Kegel area muscles, the pubococcygeal group.

If you wish to add difficulty to the maneuver, twist both legs to the left and right, tapping each handle, then return them to the center, and slowly lower them down.

You may also perform a hanging jackknife by bending at your hip fold and lifting your legs in a straight position.

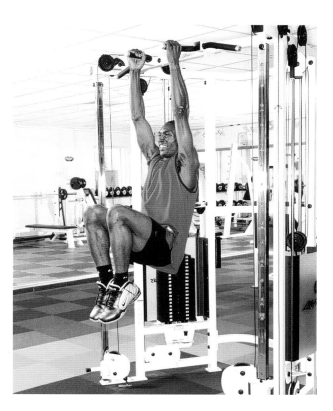

End position: Your spine should be relaxed and elongated with your feet hanging down.

Be aware: The most important precaution is to be sure your shoulders remain seated and down. You will have to make an effort to accomplish this, because the suspensory rack places the stress of your body weight directly upon your forearms and ultimately your shoulders. Relax your abdomen and breathe deeply to gain full benefit from the stretching effect upon your legs. Be certain not to "whip" your legs up and down; instead, make deliberate and slow movements.

Intermediate: Squeeze and lift a Swiss ball between your legs.

Advanced: Squeeze and lift a medicine ball between your legs.

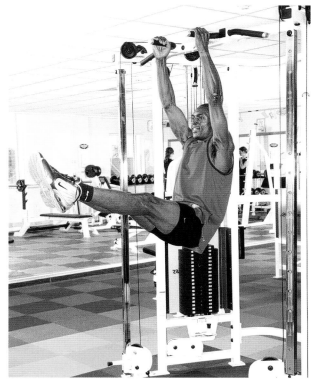

Medicine Ball

Trunk Rotation

Level: Intermediate

Suitable for: Healthy individuals, elite athletes

Area of Concentration: TA, oblique, low back

Medicine balls come in a variety of sizes and weights, depending upon the manufacturer, but they all require a degree of caution. They look innocent enough, but if you aren't ready for the weight you can strain your spine very easily. In general, hold the ball close to your trunk to avoid straining your shoulders or spine. You don't have to be an elite athlete to benefit from this training. Remember to protect your spine by keeping it actively elongated and in the correct alignment. Attention to detail is far more important than repetition. Stop before you feel discomfort, take a day of rest, then try some more.

Starting Position: Seat yourself comfortably upon a mat with your spine stretched long and the crest of your head reaching to the ceiling. Legs are flat against the mat and you are holding the medicine ball with two hands parallel on the side, about a forearm's length from your chest. The holding of the ball should feel as if it is originating from your solar plexus, a point in the middle of your trunk. To help create this feeling, press down in your armpits and keep your shoulders pressed down and open.

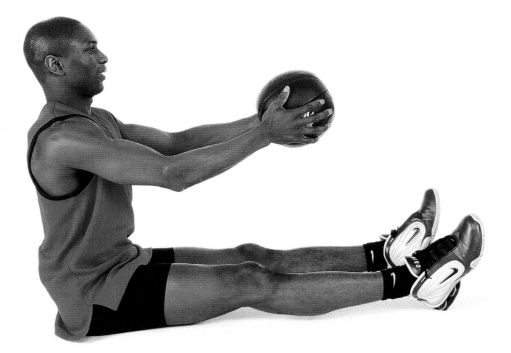

Step By Step: Begin by twisting to the right side slowly. As you twist, roll the medicine ball so that your left hand is on top and hold that position briefly on the right before slowly twisting back to the center and bringing your hand position back to parallel on the side of the ball.

Now twist to the left hand side and slowly roll the ball so that your right hand is on top. Hold that position briefly before slowly moving back to center with hand position parallel.

Repeat this eight times, slowly.

Ending Position: The medicine ball is brought to rest in your lap as you sit with your spine straight on the mat.

Be Aware: Remember that you must keep your shoulders in a seated position with your spine long. The slow movement is borrowed from power movements in T'ai Chi forms, and it is meant to impose discipline upon the strengthening action.

Relax your abdomen and breathe deeply to gain full benefit from the stretching effect upon your legs.

Advanced: You may perform this exercise while seated on a Swiss ball.

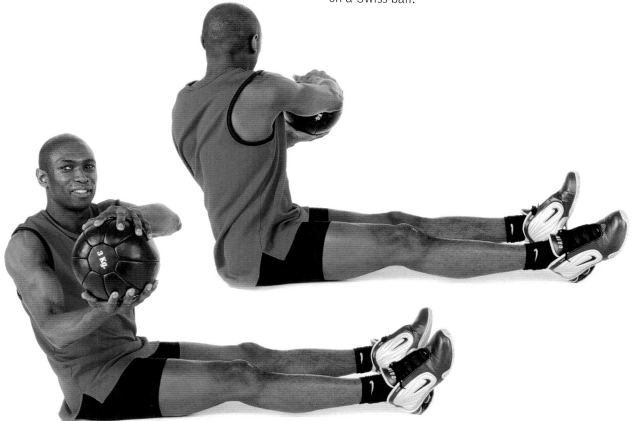

Leg Raise

Level: Advanced

Suitable for: Elite athletes

Area of Concentration: Abdominals, iliopsoas

Once you have mastered simple leg raises and leg raises with twists, you are ready to make it more difficult. Adding some weight to the equation will strengthen the iliopsoas and abdominals even further.

You are supporting your entire body weight upon both forearms, which can create unnatural strain in your shoulders. If you do feel stress in your rotator cuff or shoulders in general, there are plenty of mat-based alternatives available. In the absence of a suspensory rack, you may use a hanging bar to improvise the situation where your legs hand freely.

Start position: Mount the suspensory rack by resting both forearms on the pads and pressing gently with your lower spine against the padded back support. Your spine should be extended as straight as possible, while your legs hang freely. Have a partner help you position a medicine ball between your knees in preparation for your exercise.

Exercise: Bend from your hip joints as you lift your knees towards your chest. You should experience a flexing sensation at the point where your leg joins your core body. Be sure to keep your hips rolled under and do not allow your lower spine to arch. Hold that position, then slowly release the legs back to the straight-down position. While completing the repetition, remember also to contract your Kegel area muscles, the pubococcygeal group, while squeezing together with your knees. Do eight repetitions, then

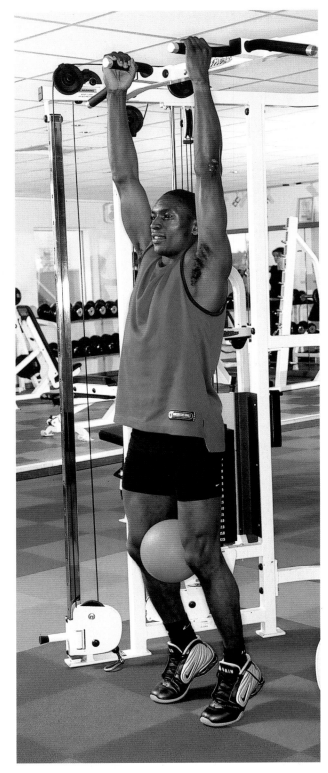

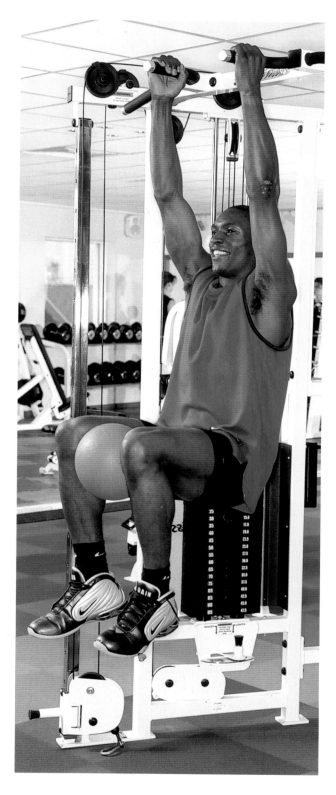

repeat the exercise with the medicine ball between your ankles. If you wish to add difficulty to the maneuver, twist both legs to the left and right, tapping each handle, then return them to the center and slowly lower them down.

End position: Keep your spine relaxed and elongated and your feet hanging down.

Be aware: The most important precaution is to be sure your shoulders remain seated and down. You will have to make an effort to accomplish this, because the suspensory rack places the stress of your body weight directly upon your forearms and ultimately your shoulders. Relax your abdomen and breathe deeply to gain full benefit from the stretching effect upon your legs. Be certain not to "whip" your legs up and down; instead, make deliberate and slow movements.

Alternative: You may perform this exercise using a small Swiss ball.

Alternative/advanced: You may add difficulty by adding a twist in between the leg lifts. If you want even more resistance, you may add ankle weights.

Russian Twist

Level: Intermediate
Suitable for: Healthy individuals, elite athletes
Area of Concentration: Abdominals, obliques

The trunk rotation exercises help you to develop oblique tone and power. Performing a twist under the duress of static abdominal contraction brings much more tone to the core, while encouraging flexibility in your erector spinae.

Protect your spine by keeping it elongated. Attention to detail is far more important than repetition. Stop before you feel discomfort.

Start position: Seat yourself comfortably upon a mat with your spine elongated and the crest of head reaching to the ceiling. Bend your legs at the knee, forming a 90-degree angle, and hold the medicine ball with two hands parallel on the side about a forearm's length from your chest. Hold the ball so that it feels as if it is originating from your solar plexus, a point in the middle of your trunk. To help create this feeling, press down in your armpits and keep your shoulders pressed down and open.

Exercise: Begin by slowly lowering yourself backward to a 45-degree angle off the ground. Twist to the right while holding that position. As you twist, roll the medicine ball so that your left hand is on top. Hold that position briefly on the right before slowly twisting back to the center and bringing your hands back to a parallel position on the side of the ball.

Now twist to the left-hand side and slowly roll the ball so that your right hand is on top. Hold that position briefly before slowly moving back to center with your hands parallel. Repeat this eight times

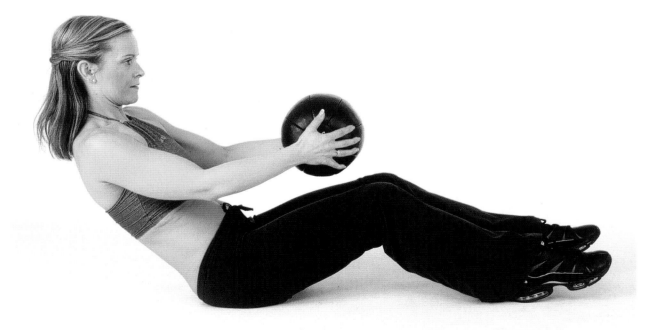

slowly. When you have mastered the exercise with your feet on the ground, try it with legs extended straight and held at 45-degree angle.

End position: The medicine ball is brought to rest in your lap as you sit with your spine straight on the mat.

Be aware: Remember that you must keep your shoulders in a seated position with your spine elongated. The slow movement is meant to impose discipline upon the strengthening action.

Relax your abdomen and breathe deeply to gain full benefit from the stretching effect upon your legs.

Advanced: You may perform this exercise with heavier medicine balls and hold the legs extended at a 45-degree angle off the mat.

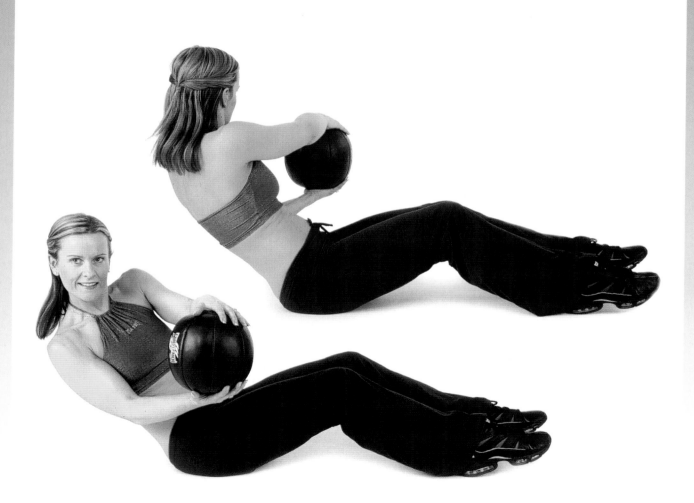

Trunk Rotation

Level: Advanced

Suitable for: Healthy individuals, athletes

Area of concentration: Abdominals, obliques

After trying trunk rotations with the medicine ball seated on the ground, why not introduce a degree of variability. By sitting on top of a Swiss ball, you activate the gluteals, iliopsoas and the erector spinalis

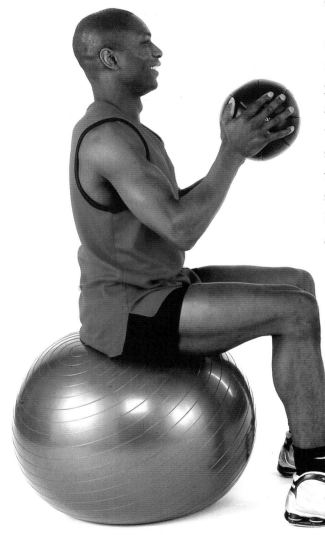

as you constantly readjust to remain on the ball. Stabilizing your trunk weight during movement of the weighted medicine ball offers a chance to tone your whole core.

Again, this exercise is not only for the elite, but you ought to be prepared and have a strong core basis. Protect your spine by keeping it elongated and actively stretching. Attention to detail is far more important than repetition. Stop before you feel discomfort, take a day of rest, then try some more.

Start position: Seat yourself comfortably upon the Swiss ball with your spine elongated and the crest of your head reaching to the ceiling. Keep your feet flat against the mat or anchored against a wall and hold the medicine ball with your two hands parallel on the side, about a forearm's length from your chest. Hold the ball so that it feels as if it is originating from your solar plexus, a point in the middle of your trunk. To help create this feeling, press down in your armpits, and keep your shoulders pressed down and open.

Exercise: Roll your hips under and elongate your spine one more time. Begin by twisting to the right side slowly. As you twist, roll the medicine ball so that your left hand is on top and hold that position briefly on the right before slowly twisting back to the center and bringing your hands back to parallel on the side of the ball.

Now twist to the left hand side and slowly roll the ball so that your right hand is on top. Hold that position briefly before slowly moving back to center with your hands parallel. Repeat this eight times slowly.

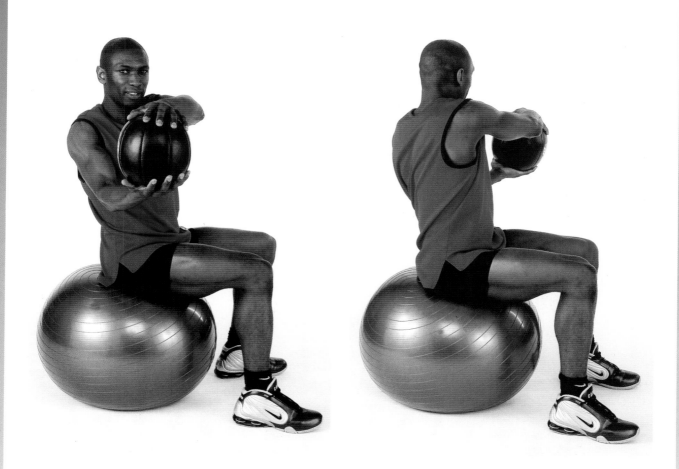

End position: The medicine ball is brought to rest on your lap as you sit on the Swiss ball.

Be aware: Remember that you must keep your shoulders in a seated position with your spine elongated. The slow movement is meant to impose discipline upon the strengthening action. Relax your abdomen and breathe deeply to gain full benefit from the stretching effect upon your legs.

Alternative/advanced: Gradually increase the medicine ball weight.

Trunk-originated Lift

Level: Advanced

Suitable for: Healthy individuals, athletes

Area of concentration: Spine, TA

While still seated on the Swiss ball with your favorite medicine ball in hand, you can really test your core capabilities and tone with this exercise. You can surprise yourself with the extent to which a movement which seems to be arm-based really accentuates the muscles of your spine.

By sitting on top of the Swiss ball, you activate gluteals, iliopsoas and the erector spinalis as you constantly readjust to remain on the ball. Stabilizing your trunk weight during movement of the weighted medicine ball offers a chance to tone your whole core.

Again, this exercise is not only for the elite, but you ought to be prepared and have a strong core basis. Protect your spine by keeping it elongated and actively stretching. Think of your shoulders as deeply seated and connected to your trunk for this exercise. Stop before you feel discomfort, take a day of rest, then try some more.

Start position: Seat yourself comfortably upon the Swiss ball with your spine elongated and the crest of your head reaching to the ceiling. Keep your feet flat against the mat or anchored against a wall and holding the medicine ball with two hands parallel on the side, about a forearm's length from your chest. Hold the ball as if it is originating from your solar plexus, a point in the middle of your trunk. To help create this feeling, press down in your armpits and keep your shoulders pressed down and open.

Exercise: Breathe out as you lift the medicine ball straight up from your chest area without allowing your shoulders to shrug up or lift. Feel as if the effort is originating from your solar plexus and press only as far as your arms comfortably allow. Slowly release the press, relax the abdomen and breathe in as you bring the ball back down. Try this eight times.

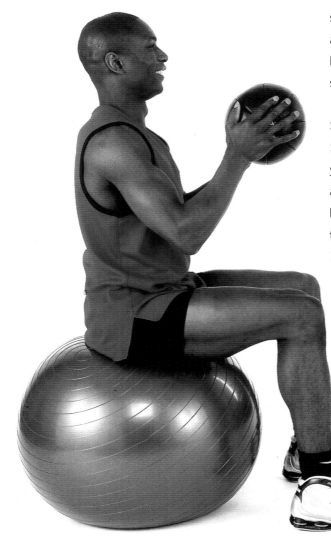

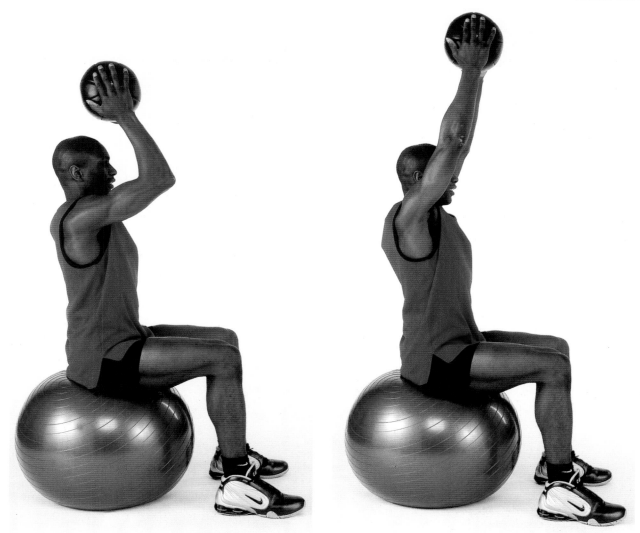

Next, try lifting the ball straight arm style. This can be very challenging for those with tender lower backs, so be very careful. Create an arc with your straight arms from your solar plexus level to over your head, always remembering to press your scapulae into your back and keep your shoulders low. Bring the ball back down to chest level.

If in doubt as to whether you feel stress in your lower spine or shoulder area, skip this altogether. Repeat this eight times slowly.

End position: Bring the medicine ball to rest on your lap as you sit on the Swiss ball.

Be aware: Remember that you must keep your shoulders in a seated position with your spine elongated. Breathe out during the extension and breathe in when returning to the original position.

Alternative/advanced: Gradually increase the weight of the medicine ball.

Partner Rotational Tosses

Level: Intermediate

Suitable for: Healthy individuals, athletes

Area of concentration: TA, obliques, erector spinae

Once you have become comfortable with the heft of a medicine ball, why not grab a partner and have some fun. Partner toss exercises are great once a good basis of core strength has been established. It is advisable to choose a partner whose training objectives, relative strength and judgment are similar to yours.

Once you start tossing around heavy objects, you enter a whole new realm of possible tears, pulls, and strains. Exercise with caution. Have fun, but remember your fundamentals. Breathe, keep your spine elongated, and allow your core muscles to do the work, not your shoulders. In general, catch the ball close to your trunk so as not to strain your shoulders or your spine. The trunk rotation exercises help you to develop oblique tone and power. However, as with all the core exercises, you derive benefits systemically. Your whole core and appendages become engaged in the activity.

Start position: Seat yourself comfortably upon a mat with your spine elongated and the crest of your head reaching to the ceiling. Your partner should do the same, facing you, with about 6 feet (2m) between both torsos. Bend your legs at 90 degrees and rest your feet against the mat. Hold the medicine ball with your two hands parallel on the side about a forearm's length from your chest.

Exercise: Begin by tossing the ball to the right side of your partner. Your partner will catch the ball by absorbing its momentum and twisting with the incoming force, then whipping the ball back to your left side. At this point, you are free to explore variation.

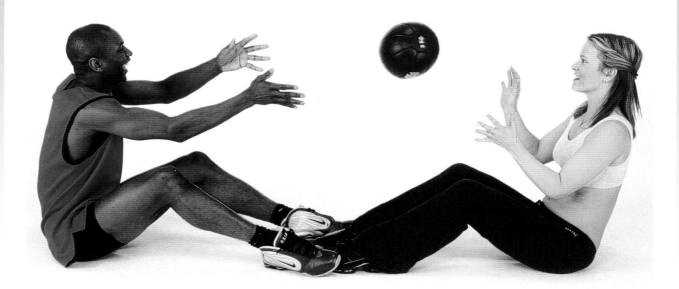

Obviously, you may continue to toss to each other on the same side. You may alternate to the opposite side or throw across the body. You may also play random, meaning that you follow no specific pattern and require your partner to be ready for whatever surprise you throw. In general, try to be accurate with the toss by keeping it close to the side. Wide throws create more strain on the shoulders and spine. A toss directly at the body requires absorbing the incoming momentum for the catch, which works the abdominals more than the obliques. You may attempt 20 repetitions for this exercise. You may also choose to perform this exercise while standing. The spacing and positional guidelines still apply. Make sure that your standing posture is solid and relaxed, with your feet shoulder width apart, toes facing each other, and hips tucked under. Your core absorbs the momentum of the ball in all instances.

End position: The medicine ball is brought to rest in your lap as you sit with your spine straight on the mat.

Be aware: Remember that you must keep your shoulders in a seated position with your spine elongated. The slow movement is meant to impose discipline upon the strengthening action.

Relax your abdomen and breathe deeply to gain full benefit from the stretching effect upon your legs.

Alternative/advanced: You may perform this exercise while standing.

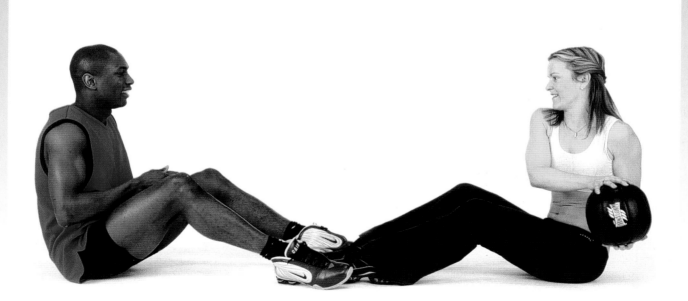

Partner Thruster Tosses

Level: Advanced

Suitable for: Healthy individuals, athletes

Area of concentration: Abdominals, lower spine

Direct partner toss exercises such as this are terrific for overall core dynamism, but a good basis of core strength has to be established in advance. It is advisable to choose a partner whose training objectives, relative strength, and judgment is similar to yours. As mentioned earlier, once you start tossing around heavy objects, you enter a whole new realm of possible tears, pulls, and strains. Exercise with caution. Have fun, but remember your fundamentals. Breathe, keep your spine elongated, and allow your core muscles to do the work, not your shoulders.

Start position: Seat yourself comfortably upon a mat with your spine elongated and the crest of your head reaching to the ceiling. Your partner will do the same, facing you, with about 6 feet (2m) between both torsos. Legs are bent 90 degrees and feet rest against the mat. Hold the medicine ball with your two hands parallel on the side, about a forearm's length from your chest.

Exercise: Begin by tossing the ball at your partner's chest. Your partner should catch the ball by absorbing its momentum and reclining until his or her shoulder blades tap the mat. The force of the throw should feel as if it came form your solar plexus, and your shoulders should be seated.

Now you must prepare for a toss back as your partner contracts the abdomen muscles, sits back up and flings the ball with both hands toward your chest. The relative force used in tossing the ball back and forth is a negotiated topic amongst partners.

You may also choose to perform this exercise with one partner standing. The spacing and positional guidelines still apply. Make sure that your standing posture is solid and relaxed, with feet shoulder width apart, toes facing each other, and hips tucked under. Your core absorbs the momentum of the ball in all instances, and your partner still aims for the chest so that you may absorb the throw with your abs.

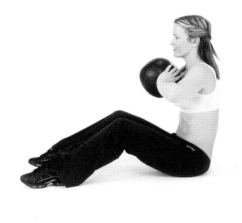

End position: The medicine ball is brought to rest in your lap as you sit with your spine straight on the mat.

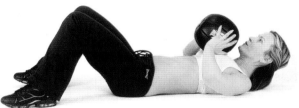

Be aware: Remember that you must keep your shoulders in a seated position with your spine elongated. Relax your abdomen and breathe deeply to gain full benefit from the stretching effect upon your legs.

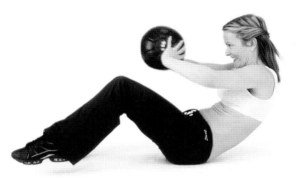

Alternative/advanced: You may perform this exercise with heavier medicine balls.

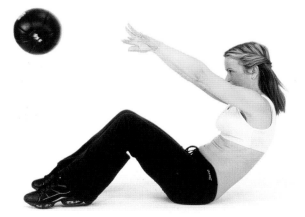

Partner Twisting Handoffs

Level: Intermediate
Suitable for: Healthy individuals, athletes

The Twisting Handoff is another example of an exercise that allows you to challenge yourself and have fun with your partner. See who moves faster. Pick up the tempo on this one without losing alignment.

Again, exercise with caution. Have fun, but remember your fundamentals. Breathe, keep your spine elongated, and allow your core muscles to do the work, not your shoulders. In general, keep the ball relatively close to your trunk.

The trunk rotation exercises help you to develop oblique tone and power. However, as with all the core exercises, you derive benefits systemically. Your whole core and appendages become engaged in the activity.

Start position: Seat yourself comfortably upon a mat with your spine elongated and the crest of your head reaching to the ceiling. Your partner sits back-to-back with you, allowing for one medicine ball's worth of spacing between you. Bend your legs 90 degrees and rest your feet against the mat. Hold the medicine ball with your two hands parallel on the side, about a forearm's length from your chest.

Exercise: Begin by turning to your right side and handing the ball to your partner. Immediately turn around to your left side in order to receive the ball back from your partner, then bring the ball around to your right side again, keeping it low and a forearm's length away from your chest. Repeat ten times then reverse direction, noticing whether you or your partner is quicker getting around for the next handoff. Take the opportunity to tease your partner if you are faster.

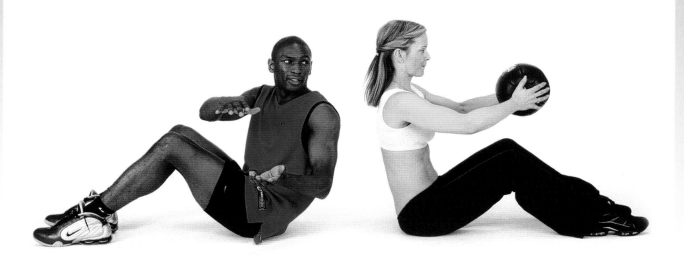

You may also choose to perform this exercise while standing. The spacing and positional guidelines still apply. Make sure that your standing posture is solid and relaxed, with your feet shoulder width apart and hips tucked under. Your core absorbs the momentum of the ball in all instances.

End position: The medicine ball is dropped to the ground because by now you should be exhausted.

Be aware: Remember that you must keep your shoulders in a seated position with your spine elongated. If you are having trouble with your shoulders creeping up, press down in the armpits. Relax your abdomen and breathe deeply to gain full benefit from the stretching effect upon your legs.

Advanced: You may perform this exercise while standing.

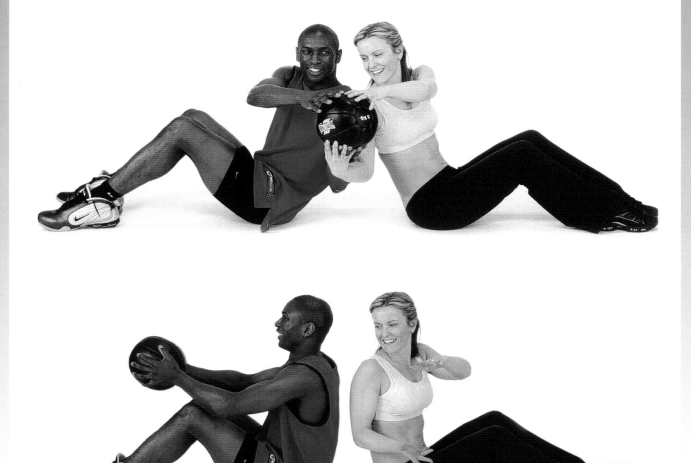

Warm Down

Warm Down Twists

Level: All

Suitable for: Healthy individuals

Unsuitable for: Back injuries

Area of concentration: Erector spinalis, abdominals, full core

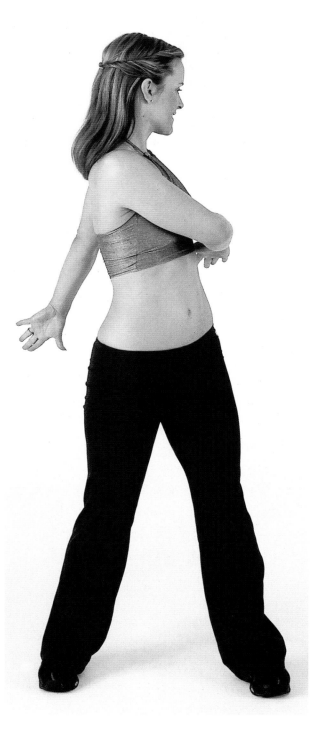

Regardless of the level of vigorous or concentrated activity, it is always good to end with twisting, easy warm down movements.

These twists allow for relaxed and subtle weight shift, easy torso movement, and good encouragement for circulation. Following a workout which may at times have called for severe and strenuous muscle contractions and concentrated effort, you need to shake off tightness and begin the easy transition to the next part of your day.

When warming your body for exercise, the initial aim is to raise heart rate and body temperature without forcing abrupt change upon bodily tissue. You can stress your tissues during exercise, so it is essential to warm down.

This Daoist-inspired twisting motion from T'ai Chi Chuan induces a feeling of blood flow to stimulate the carriage of nutrients to every cell in the body and the exchange of the byproducts of extreme effort (lactic acids, proteins, etc.) out of the body. Every body type is different, so every person will "warm up" and "warm down" at a different rate and with a different style. However, it is important that we all slowly adjust our core temperature with basic movement back to a normal functioning level.

Start position: Place your feet slightly wider than shoulder width apart. Focus your eyes forward. Relax your arms at your side, and begin by imagining your spine as a straight cylindrical column.

Tuck your chin in and lift your head toward the ceiling from its crown. Imagine you are being stretched upward by a rope attached to the crown of your skull. Allow your knees to flex and roll your hips under as you imagine the southern tip of your spine being pulled down by an attached weight. Open the hips so that the knees are vertically in line with the feet. Press forward at the fold of the hip joint, which is actually located at the front of the pelvis where your leg meets your trunk.

Relax your facial muscles and keep your shoulders "seated" as you press down in your armpits. Press down in your armpits to seat the shoulders in a natural position so that levator muscles are not tugging them upward toward your head and tightening vertebrae along the way.

Pressing down in the armpits helps you to engage the effort necessary to elongate the spine upward. In the area of the Thoracic (upper) vertebrae, imagine a stretch upward. In the area of the lumbar (lower) vertebrae, imagine a stretch down to the ground. Our scapula—the bones at the end of each arm that integrate with the back muscles—should be relaxed and flush with the back and feel "open," pressing forward into the back. You should feel no pinching of the scapula toward each other.

Exercise: Begin your twists by slowly rotating our spine, a straight column, back and forth, imagining our whole body rotating around a central vertical axis. Dangle your arms loosely by your side and concentrate on the feeling of balance in your feet. Allow your arms

to follow your waist as it twists slightly faster. However, never lead the movement of your core body with arm action. The arms should follow your core as they work your large internal musculature.

End position: Slow your rotation and return to a standing posture, your feet slightly wider than shoulder width apart. Tuck your hips under, flexing your knees, and tuck your chin in to keep your spine elongated. Breathe in a relaxed manner through your nose with each distinct contraction and release your abdomen muscles with each expansion and contraction of your rib cage.

Be aware: The twisting movement comes from turning the waist back and forth around the axis of the spine. Do not force the twist with surface muscles. Feel it come from your core.

Conclusion

You have now worked through a good selection of the many exercise variations you might experience in core training.

For all ages and all abilities, core training is a safe and effective way to improve the body's capabilities and encourage better health. Start your program today. Every step you take toward a stronger and more flexible core means a step towards better fitness. Core training integrates all your physical activity, so you will notice results rapidly. When your core is stronger and more flexible, you feel better, look better, and will use your body more effectively. Who could argue with core training for greater strength and better health?

Index